Richard A. Hughes

The Radiant Shock of Death

PETER LANG
New York • Washington, D.C./Baltimore • San Francisco
Bern • Frankfurt am Main • Berlin • Vienna • Paris

Library of Congress Cataloging-in-Publication Data

Hughes, Richard.
　　The radiant shock of death / Richard A. Hughes.
　　　　p.　　cm. — (American university studies. Series VII, Theology and religion; vol. 183)
　　Includes bibliographical references and index.
　　1. Death—Religious aspects—Christianity.　2. Death—Psychological aspects.　3. Thanatology.　I. Title.　II. Series.
BT825.H845.　　　　　　　　236'.1—dc20　　　　　　　　94-25330
ISBN 0-8204-2610-5
ISSN 0740-0446

Die Deutsche Bibliothek-CIP-Einheitsaufnahme

Hughes, Richard A.:
The radiant shock of death / Richard A. Hughes. - New York; Washington, D.C./Baltimore; San Francisco; Bern; Frankfurt am Main; Berlin; Vienna; Paris: Lang.
　　(American university studies: Ser. 7, Theology and religion; Vol. 183)
　　ISBN 0-8204-2610-5
NE: American university studies / 02

The paper in this book meets the guidelines for permanence and durability of the Committee on Production Guidelines for Book Longevity of the Council on Library Resources.

Printed in the United States of America.

The Radiant Shock of Death

American University Studies

Series VII
Theology and Religion
Vol. 183

PETER LANG
New York • Washington, D.C./Baltimore • San Francisco
Bern • Frankfurt am Main • Berlin • Vienna • Paris

In Memory of

My Father and Mother

William and Dorothy Hughes

ACKNOWLEDGMENT

For the preparation of this book I am indebted to several persons. David Hufford of the Hershey Medical School provided a few sources on bereavement visionary phenomena. Howard Kee of the University of Pennsylvania identified key shock terms in the Greek text of the Gospel of Mark. The British analyst Albert Hughes, who by the way is not related to me, helped clarify the relationships between Sigmund Freud, Carl Jung, and Leopold Szondi. Janet Hurlbert, Cheryl Yearick, and Marlene Neece of the Snowden Library at Lycoming College collected many bibliographical materials. I gratefully acknowledge the contributions of these colleagues.

Unless otherwise stated, biblical quotations are taken from the New Revised Standard Version of the Bible, copyright 1989, by the Division of Christian Education of the National Council of the Churches of Christ in the USA and are used with permission. Translations of French, German, and Greek sources are my own, and responsibility for any errors of translation or interpretation is also mine. My wife Diane prepared the manuscript for publication, and my daughter Heather helped type the references.

Some of the materials in chapters three, seven, and eight were presented orally in the Szondi Prize Lecture, entitled "The Symbolism of the Bridge" and delivered at the University of Zürich on June 18, 1993. I am profoundly grateful to Ralf Krek, Mary Spreng, and Fritz Stolz, who spoke publically on behalf of my work. While in Zürich, I had stimulating dialogue with Friedjung Jüttner and Karl Bürgi-Meyer at the Szondi Institut. Hanny Mouche also served as a gracious hostess for me, my wife, and my children.

TABLE OF CONTENTS

PREFACE

Three experiences have compelled me to write this book. First, I teach Death and Dying every semester, every academic year, and sometimes in special sessions. Except for sabbatical leaves, I have taught this course continuously since 1973. The students enrolled in the course represent all fields in the liberal arts curriculum. Many have had dramatic death experiences, which they bring to the course either openly, privately, or described through written assignments. These experiences usually involve symbolic forms, such as dreams and religious questions, which tend to be neglected in society and the health care professions. For example, as I write this preface, an experienced nurse-student has raised a typical question. Her dying patient dreams of fires breaking out and burning all over her. What do these fires mean, she asks? In light of the theory advanced in this book fire symbolizes pent-up emotion and the need for restitution.

My concern as a pastorally-oriented teacher is to interpret death symbols and to integrate these into a clinically-grounded body of knowledge. Generally, textbooks are not sufficiently interdisciplinary. They are written primarily by psychiatrists or psychologists who, though well trained in clinical methods, lack broad knowledge, particularly in the history of religions. Religious traditions are frequently decisive in shaping the symbolic forms of death experiences.

As an example, I offer an anecdotal illustration. On March 8, 1992 I received a telephone call from a former school-mate of mine who was an AIDS patient. I asked if he had any dreams, and he said yes. In the dream he is standing in a ditch along side a country road, and a halo encompasses his head. A friend, standing on the road above is calling for him to return, but he remains in the ditch.

Immediately, I recognized this to be a death dream, and I knew he would die soon. Descent to the ditch is a death image, reflecting the old Hebrew conception of Sheol. The halo signifies radiant being and acceptance of death. The country road reenacts the pre-Christian practice of burying the dead outside the city. The refusal to go back to the road indicates that the AIDS patient has become a stranger, alienated from society. Sadly but not surprisingly, I learned some time later that he died on September 18, 1992.

Pioneers in death studies have broken through traditional organic approaches in psychiatry and established psychosocial models of dying and bereavement. They have shown that death experiences are unique and not reducible to general psychiatry or psychology. Avery Weisman has contributed analyses of denial and its variants, types of coping, the role of relationships in illness, and the concept of an appropriate death (1974). Elisabeth Kübler-Ross has conceptualized five consecutive stages of dying: (1) denial and isolation, (2) anger, (3) bargaining, (4) depression, and (5) acceptance (1969). These have caught on in the public mind and have helped shape a popular death culture. They have also informed local hospice and bereavement support groups.

However, the Kübler-Ross theory of stages presents a teaching problem in the sense that it has never been revised or verified by other clinicians. In her book on AIDS she indicates that the notion of stages is an older concept and now to be regarded as a theory of emotional reactions, expressed by patients, families, and professional care-givers (Kübler-Ross 1987, 1). She insists that these reactions recur, over and over again, but not in any "chronological order." Yet she continues to discuss them, as though they were in a prescribed order.

A definitive assessment has been made by Robert Kastenbaum (1991, 102). He argues convincingly that the Kübler-Ross theory is prescriptive not descriptive, subjective not objective. Her stages represent ideals rather than universal patterns. In fact, when care-givers concentrate on stages, they tend to ignore other aspects of dying, such as the patient's biography or family background. Dying is personal, and its uniqueness may not be expressed in stages but in symbolic language, dreams, and leave-taking rituals. Kastenbaum's critique illustrates the fact that a theory of terminal illness, narrowly construed, does not provide a framework to integrate familial and symbolic forms. One reason for my writing this book is to integrate clinical symbolism with patient decision making and familial relatedness. So-called stages are herein regarded as defenses, which occur but not in any order.

Kübler-Ross defines her mission as helping professional care-givers and the clergy to appreciate the needs of the dying. As a member of the clergy, I express my profound gratitude to her life and work, her caring and courage, but I am troubled by her "theological" judgments. She states that negativity is the enemy of life, and since negativity depletes energy, it should be removed in order to provide acceptance in death. Negativity comprises fear, guilt, and shame, emotions that are excluded from her stage theory. Elimination of these affects is justified by her notion of "divine manipulation" and represented in the following rule: "You always get what you need at the right time" (Kübler-Ross 1987,

194). She defends her point of view in the context of Christianity and the life of Jesus.

Certainly, her idea of "divine manipulation" invites a theological criticism, specifically that her idea of acceptance is a regression to a primary narcissism (Miller-McLemore 1988, 96). Acceptance of death as narcissistic fulfillment of wishing can neither dissolve opposites nor remove negativity, because narcissism itself is a defense against death. Christianity approaches the problem of death from the radical negativism of the crucifixion of Jesus. The crucifixion is a terrible shock-event, bringing total darkness and threatening complete abandonment. Consequently, the concluding three chapters of this book develop a theology of death that accounts for extreme dread, unmanageable pain, and despair.

The second motive for writing this book is my long-time study of the life and work of Leopold Szondi, the eminent Hungarian-born, Swiss psychiatrist. Since he is not well known in the United States, I wrote my previous book as an introduction to his thought (Hughes 1992). This book develops ideas, which would have exceeded the scope of that volume.

One of Szondi's major contributions is his concept of the familial unconscious. This idea grew out of his early scientific research in Budapest, begun in 1927 and ended in 1944 when the Nazi Party imprisoned him in Bergen-Belsen Concentration Camp. The familial unconscious carries genetic traits, throughout several generations, that influence personal decision-making including the choice of death. Modes of dying are likely to be familial, that is, repetitions of tendencies latent in the genotype. These may emerge spontaneously in dreams and visions of the dying. For example, in families transmitting the "attack syndrome" of illness, descendants are at risk for sudden or shock deaths. In families with schizoform traits, members are inclined to express projective-participatory thought. While dying, this mode of thought emerges in the attempt to strip away the body and strive for an exalted spiritual participation.

Szondi was also one of the pre-eminent pioneers in the study of epilepsy. On the basis of classical psychiatry he conceptualized the paroxysmal pattern, which functions as the biological structure of the "attack syndrome." Although absent in American thought, this concept offers a coherent explanation of the varieties of shock death, including death-bed visions, near-death experiences, and the epileptic seizures of AIDS.

Closely related to the paroxysmal theory is his ego psychology, which is informed by the symbolism of the bridge. The bridge motif symbolizes the unification of opposites through basic decision-making and is frequently found in visions of death among the religions of the world. When the bridge symbol appears in shock events, it means that negativity is raised to a transpersonal spiritual state. The bridge symbol properly illustrates the fact that negativity does not go away but becomes transformed.

The third and most compelling reason for writing this book is the death of my parents. My story of their deaths begins in November, 1973, six weeks before my wedding in December. I had a series of dreams, consisting of two types. In one a bridge spanned a large body of water. A man and a woman walked across the bridge from the near shore to the farther shore. In the other a man and a woman rode in a boat across a large lake, amid several islands, and landed on the distant shore. I interpreted both types of dreams as unconscious projections of my unfolding destiny. They told me that my marriage choice was appropriate, and our relationship was whole.

However, I had an overwhelming sense of death with these dreams, but I did not know why. About the same time as my wedding, though unknown to me, my mother was also having a series of dreams. In one she saw my father dead, lying in an open split-top casket, dressed in a blue pin-striped suit, white shirt, and red tie—exactly as he would look during his funeral. In the other she was walking in a long, dark tunnel toward a light in the distance. My father was walking ahead of her in the same tunnel. Both walked toward the light, but neither left the tunnel.

Meanwhile, sixteen years passed by. My father was a Methodist pastor, living in Indiana and struggling with heart disease. He suffered intense pain and bodily weakness throughout the summer of 1989. By October he expressed the wish to have a "dying at will," as practiced in the Hawaiian Islands. During the Thanksgiving week, he acted out unconscious "leave-taking" rituals, saying good-bye to an old friend and speaking with me in Pennsylvania on the telephone. His voice had an unusually clear quality. Although not scheduled to preach on the following Sunday, he was unexpectedly called to do so due to a near-fatal automobile accident by his ministerial colleague. So on Sunday, November 26, he entered the pulpit for the last time.

In previous years he had suffered a hearing loss and a paralyzed vocal chord that made his speaking voice harsh and raspy. While conducting the service, he became transfigured and radiated a silver aura. His speaking and hearing returned to normal clarity. His sermon text was Psalm 23, and as he expounded it he seemed to achieve a profound serenity. Departing from the text, he had a vision of crossing waters to the distant shore. Shortly after his visionary sermon, he suffered a seizure death.

When my father died, I realized the meaning of my wedding dreams. In the shock of love and death father and son chose the same symbolism—crossing the waters to the distant shore. Whether crossing by bridge or by boat, the symbolism portrayed a transfigured state of awareness, in which the antitheses of life and death were united. In marriage I achieved an essential relatedness, and in death my father attained his primal form.

My mother's 1973 dreams also foreshadowed my father's death. They were precognitive familial dreams, expressing anticipatory grief. With my father's death her grieving proceeded without complication. She accepted his death, moved to Pennsylvania, and built an addition onto our house for her new residence.

Shortly after burying my father in Pennsylvania, psychic activity began to happen around my two children. My son Jimmy, then four years old, was suddenly frightened by a luminous presence in the early evening of December 14, 1989. My wife Diane confirmed the existence of "footstep" hauntings in the hallway between Jimmy's bedroom and my daughter Heather's, who was then eight years old. These began during the week of February 5, 1990 and usually occurred about 10:30 p.m.. On March 7, which was my mother's birthday, I heard a loud "falling" sound at four o'clock in the morning, awakening my wife and son. Thereafter, the "footstep" hauntings continued to be heard for about one year. The last haunting was witnessed on February 7, when my mother was in a local hospital. In the perspective of this book, these hauntings derived from the afterimage of my father's radiant death. Their intention was to bid farewell to his grandchildren.

My mother had been a cancer patient since 1985. She had entered the hospital on January 14, 1991 for treatment of an infection, but by Sunday, February 10, tests indicated kidney failure and imminent death.

I conferred with her oncologist concerning conditions of the cessation of treatment, as she had stipulated in her living will.

On Monday I went to the hospital in the afternoon, following my classes. When I walked into the room, she asked: "Am I dying?" I replied: "I don't know, mother." I felt that only she should answer that question. She explained that she had been dreaming of her funeral and of her death. I understood these dreams to signify a relativization of time, a clairvoyance of future events, and therefore an early phase of dying.

At six o'clock in the morning of the next day, she told her nurse: "I am dying." Since the nurse had been one of my students, she reported this declaration by telephone, and I began to grieve.

I conducted a morning class and arrived at the hospital at twelve noon. I walked into the room, and mother announced, "I'm not dead yet." I asked if she were dreaming, and she said: "All the time." Sensing an impending visionary phase, I requested a sheet of paper, sat down at the table near the bed, and recorded the following dialogue:

12:05   Richard: "Do you see father?"
         Mother: "Yes. He doesn't say anything. I see my whole life. Same thing over and over again." She stops talking and falls asleep.

12:10   M: "Don't talk to me. I know you're here. That's all that matters."

12:15   She appears half-asleep and moaning.
         M: "Let me go!" She continues to moan and, periodically, has hiccups, twitchings, shivering, and seizures.

12:30   Her throat is parched, and she sips some water.

12:40   M: "Why am I still alive?"

12:50   M: "I hear music, off and on."
         R: "Is it pretty music, mother?"
         M: "Not particularly."

12:55   She alternates between sleeping and moaning.
         M: "What? Yes."

1:25   M: "Oh, God!"

2:25   She asks for water.

2:30   She moans and chants repeatedly: "Oh, God! Help me."

2:45   M: "One more day. Oh, God!

Oh, God. Let me go!

Oh, God. Help me. I'm not dead yet."

3:00 A pastoral care nurse enters the room and asks her if she wants pain medication.

M: "No medicine."

The nurse says the Lord's Prayer and leaves the room. Meanwhile, another nurse comes into the room, stands at the bedside, and says to me that mother is hallucinating in defense against pain. I reply: "I beg your pardon. Let's go out into the hallway and talk about this." We both leave the room and stand in the corridor, as another nurse joins us. I explain that my mother is experiencing authentic death-bed visions and not hallucinations. She had just declined pain medications, because visions tend to diminish pain. Her chanting has revealed an entirely unexpected change of personality. She is now in a "split-off," visionary phase.

The nurse asks if there were any stages, and I say no. I suggest that by looking for stages, she would miss the interior spirituality, as expressed in mother's struggle to strip away the body. The nurse admits that members of her own family have had similar visions, and she thanks me for pointing them out to her.

I believe that the shock of dying has dramatically revealed two unconscious, familial tendencies in mother's "split-off" phase. First, the striving to escape the body brings out her projective-participatory mode of thought, as manifest by the psychics and Spiritualists in the maternal branch of her family. Second, the ecstasy comes out of her paroxysmal heredity, tendencies toward the "attack syndrome" in her father's branch. The ecstasy occurs in the dreaming, *deja vu,* and intellectual aura or celestial music. These are psychic equivalents of epilepsy, as discovered by the British neurosurgeon J. Hughlings Jackson.

I return to the bedside of my dying mother.

3:20   M: "Why is it taking so long?"

> 3:40   She raised her head and, in a strong voice, commands:
> "Go home, Richard."

I realized that she wanted to be alone and to protect me from the impact of her death. Since I respected her wishes and was exhausted, I went home. During the night, I spoke on the telephone several times with the nurse. I learned that the artificially delivered nutrition (TPN) was withdrawn at six o'clock in the evening. Meanwhile, her chanting continued until eleven o'clock. Altogether, her visionary phase lasted eleven hours—six hours with nutrition and five hours without. Hence, the visions were independent of physiological processes.

On Wednesday, February 13, I cancelled my classes and stayed at the hospital the entire day. Mother slept, and we had no dialogue or visions. A kidney specialist informed me that death would come soon. On the following morning, at 11:40, he slowed down the hydration. Mother asked: "Why am I so sick?" At 2:15 p.m. of the same day the doctor stopped all fluids. He told me that death would come within 48 hours. I waited in the hospital room all day.

On Friday morning I conducted one class and arrived at the hospital at ten o'clock. Mother was alert and speaking occasionally:

> 10:30   M: "I'm sick."
> 10:50   M: "Oh, God."
> 11:15   I walk out of the room and see one of the nurses, then off-duty, running down the hallway toward me and crying. I ask: "M—, what are you doing here?" She answers: "The spirits are present." I reply: "Who are the spirits?" She does not answer but proceeds into the room, to the bedside, and speaks with my mother: "Dorothy, are you afraid?" Mother says no and states that she wants to be with God. The nurse runs out of the room, still crying.

I remained in the room throughout the afternoon, while mother slept. At mid-afternoon, the phone rang once. I startled, but she did not. About four o'clock, Mother awoke and said: "Go home, Richard, it's too hard on you!" I replied: "No Mother, I'll stay with you," and she said: "Okay."

On Saturday, she moaned and did not talk. Diane, Heather, and Jimmy came to say good-bye. On Sunday, February 17, she continued to moan and call out: "Oh, God." By mid-afternoon her blood pressure had fallen to 60/40. At 4:30 and 8:00 in the evening, she was given morphine. Since her vital signs were diminishing, no more morphine would be administered.

Darkness settled over the room, as I listened to mother's agonal breathing. Her respirations slowed down to fewer than twelve per minute. Two images came to me. One was an analogy with the labor of birth. She had given birth to me; and now I witnessed her struggle to leave the body of death. Her agony also reminded me of the waves of the primal sea, carrying her to the distant shore to be with God and my father. Mother reached the distant shore at six o'clock in the morning.

INTRODUCTION:
A PSYCHOLOGY OF DEATH

I. SCOPE OF THIS BOOK

The aim of this book is to develop a general theory of death as a shock event. Since death experiences are so diverse, it is necessary to delimit the notion of shock death. By shock death is meant an impact of overwhelming mortal danger, resulting in startle, immobilization, or unconsciousness. Although the idea of shock is linked to death, here it is defined broadly so as to incorporate two variations: (1) physiological shock or reduction of cardiac activity, respiration, and consciousness, and (2) psychological shock, which is understood as the discharge of emotion due to startle and culminating in death, unconsciousness, or lowered threshold of consciousness.

While this study is concerned with death and dying, it draws upon depth psychology, philosophy and theology. These disciplines converge because of the interdisciplinary nature of death experience. Depth psychology helps to reveal unconscious processes, conflicts, and symbolic language in the face of death. Inevitably, philosophy intervenes, because participants in the dying process, particularly professional care-givers, tend to make judgments as to whether symptoms, pain, or symbols and so forth are real. Theology appears to the extent that ultimate issues invariably arise in dying and mourning. Questions of ultimate meaning deal primarily with the task of resolving suffering. However, the theological framework of this study is limited to that of Christianity with special attention to Protestant theology.

Further, the notion of shock death is limited to three clinical phenomena. The first is that of dreams and visions occurring within the dying process. In ordinary clinical practice these tend to be neglected or dismissed, even though they might facilitate a resolution of suffering. Neglect or rejection takes place for two common reasons.

One is the inclination to dismiss dreams and visions as hallucinations in defense against pain. This tendency grows out of an assumption, prevailing in medicine, that reality is strictly physical, objective, linear, and quantifiable. This worldview reflects the success of medical treatment, and it also narrowly prescribes the boundary of the human being. Whatever falls out of the medical paradigm is not real and can be neither treated nor interpreted. Nevertheless, dismissals of symbolic language by professional care-givers surpass the boundaries of medicine and enter into philosophical discourse.

The other reason is the preoccupation with the stages of dying. The idea of stages in the dying process belongs to popular culture, where it satisfies a need to achieve control in the face of death. Yet, searching for the stages does not necessarily resolve suffering either but even discourages attention to the whole person, to subtle messages, and to symbolism. For example, one of my students working in a hospice program in 1989, informed me of the following situation. A man was dying, and he exclaimed: "It's light in here!" Immediately, the hospice volunteers pulled the shades over the windows, closed the curtains, and shut the door. When he said the light had gone away, they reopened the windows and the door. When the light reappeared, the volunteers' actions were the same. Apparently, the man had had a vision of light, and the volunteers mistook it as a physical sensation. By acting in terms of physicalist assumptions, they may have deprived him of a significant experience.

The second topic of this book is that of bereavement dreams and visions. In my experience, the neglect of these is more common than those of terminal illness. One reason for such neglect is the relative absence of post-funeral rituals and care-giving. Frequently, the bereaved find themselves totally alone some time after a funeral, and they begin to see the deceased in images, dreams, or visions. Such occurrences shape a private drama, often bringing consolation to the bereaved, but sometimes confusion, anxiety, or fear. Providing an interpretation of these experiences helps to resolve the grieving process. Consequently, a theory is needed to integrate bereavement dreams and visions with the shock of death.

The third clinical focus of this study is the near-death experience. This is certainly well-known and extensively documented, and so there is little need to add more data. The intent of this book is to interpret the near-death experience in relationship with the dreams and visions of death and grief. The reason is that investigations of the near-death experience, at present, are concerned with whether or not it offers proof of life after death. The near-death experience is treated as a unique and unprecedented phenomenon within the province of medicine. Consequently, medical researchers employ philosophical assumptions, stated above, and overlook the interpretations of the near-death experience within the history of culture and religion. The ahistorical context of medicine uncritically obeys religious needs for ultimate truth which are latent in popular culture. Thus, this book takes seriously historical and theological studies, which are useful in analyzing the symbolic aspects of the near-death experience.

When viewed together, the three clinical areas cited above invite an interdisciplinary inquiry. Accordingly, chapters one through three will develop a psychological theory integrating shock death and historically-transmitted symbolism. Chapters four through six will analyze dreams and visions of death and grief as well as near-death experiences in terms of their common shock capacities. Finally, chapters seven through the conclusion will formulate a theological framework, based upon biblical, historical, and constructive Christian theologies. Theological attention is limited to the death experience primarily and not to the issue of life after death.

II. THE SUBLIMINAL SELF

Since this study views shock death at the intersection of several disciplines, it is appropriate to select as a starting point one of the most original and comprehensive theories of modern times. Between 1880 and 1900 in England, the classics scholar Frederic W. H. Myers (1843-1901) studied a wide range of death experiences, including claims of so-called psychic events. He was assisted by other scholars at Cambridge University, such as the philosopher Henry Sidgwick, who founded the Society for Psychical Research in 1882. While Sidgwick, along with Edmund Gurney, pursued convincing evidence for survival of biological death, Myers produced a vast synthesis of knowledge in his great work entitled **Human Personality and Its Survival of Bodily Death** (1903/1954).

Anyone who reads Myers' two volume work will readily appreciate his great visionary power, lyrical style, and rich case materials, closely analyzed and integrated in a comprehensive theory. The pivotal concept of his system is that of the subliminal self. While his scientific data and concepts need to be up-dated, his basic theory remains tenable and applicable to the notion of shock death. The remainder of this section presents a condensed summary of Myers' position, as background for his psychology of death.

Beginning with volume one, Myers acknowledges that traditionally Christianity has governed knowledge of death and access to life after death. However, in modern times some new, alternative approaches had appeared. One was trance mediumship, a movement claiming to contact spirits of the dead and becoming quite popular in the late nineteenth century. Myers also notes that one of the intellectual predecessors, in the eighteenth century, was the Swedish engineer and mystic Emanuel Swedenborg. At age 55, Swedenborg began to suffer a series of seizures which, he alleged, opened up contact with the spirits of deceased persons. He purported to be in communication with the spirit world for 30 years. Myers states that Swedenborg conceived of the invisible other world as a realm of law (I, 6). If his experiences were authentic, as Myers suspects they were, then the other world ought to be accessible to scholarly exploration.

The law of the other world, which Myers seeks to prove, is that of telepathy, which he defines as communication from mind to mind outside ordinary sensory channels (I, 8). As the fundamental law of motion in the other world, telepathy corresponds to that of gravity in the physical universe. Myers finds that in times of danger or death telepathy intensifies and behaves in the manner of gravity, that is, as a wave-like field of attraction. He and his colleagues collected extensive data to document the working of telepathy. However, Myers could not easily move from data to proof, particularly, as it relates to life after death; so he developed the theory of the subliminal self to account for a psychology of death. With the notion of the subliminal self Myers became the first scholar in the English speaking world to conceive of the unconscious.

The subliminal self contains levels of awareness, beginning with ordinary waking consciousness in the bodily ego. Waking consciousness is transitory, unstable, and susceptible to breaks of attention. The ego relies on sense organs to acquire information from the external world of objects. The senses function like filters that screen out excessive stimuli; but occasionally, they rupture and allow unfiltered stimuli to overload neural channels. The workings of waking consciousness may be compared metaphorically to ripples on the surface of a sea.

A considerable range of mental activity occurs below the level of waking consciousness. A helpful analogy for the regions of the subliminal self would be the solar spectrum. Light may be visible at the center of the spectrum, but, at the ends, it turns into an invisible radiance. This spectrum analogy illumines the fact that an extensive continuum of consciousness co-exists with the physical universe. This latter aspect is the subliminal self, and its relationship with waking consciousness involves a threshold. Consciousness "above" the threshold is called supraliminal and that "below" subliminal. Both supraliminal and subliminal selves act together and comprise a complementary whole. However, the subliminal self can generate impulses that take over the threshold and release upheavals within the consciousness.

Myers took over the idea of threshold from the nineteenth century studies of hysteria. During the 1880s, Pierre Janet, Joseph Breuer, and Sigmund Freud observed that the mental threshold underlying waking consciousness can be raised and lowered. It is unstable and, under certain conditions, the mental threshold might be lowered to the degree of unconsciousness or dissociation. Janet conceived of the threshold in the context of hypnotism, which the new French psychiatry advocated along with Jean Charcot. Breuer and Freud, working in Vienna, discovered the instability of the mental threshold in terms of hysteria. Whereas Janet attributed a lowered threshold to a congenital failure of the capacity for mental synthesis, Freud argued that it was due to unconscious conflict caused by repression of a dynamic impulse.

To a certain extent, Myers' explanation of a lowered threshold was similar to Freud's. Myers held that unconscious impulses would erupt, take over the personality and create a loss of consciousness or splitting. Portions of the subliminal self can break out, split apart, and penetrate waking consciousness as fixed idea-forces. These conditions of dissociation are convulsive, and not reducible to repression, and they involve a wide range of seizure activities, including hysteria but, especially, epilepsy. As indicated by Myers' chapter titles, the range comprises the following list: (1) disintegration (e.g., hysteria, epilepsy);

(2) genius; (3) sleep; (4) hypnotism; (5) sensory automatism; (6) phantasms of the dead; (7) motor automatism; and (8) trance, possession and ecstasy. Appended to each of these topics is an extensive collection of cases. However, implied in this list is Myers' contention that dissociation states are not abnormal but are means of creativity and transcendent ecstasy, as well as telepathy.

Dissociative states are creative because of the fundamental continuity of mind in itself. Despite mental upheavals, the supraliminal and subliminal selves retain a relationship. This continuity of mind parallels the hierarchical structure of the brain (I, 72). A contemporary of Myers, J. Hughlings Jackson discovered the tripartite structure of the brain in his studies of epilepsy. He conceived of higher cortical levels, controlling thought and will; and a middle level as the source of muscular movements; and lower levels, governing automatic processes like circulation and respiration. When the epileptic seizure effects the higher brain centers, then the middle range acts compulsively in a fit. Similarly, when the convulsion effects the middle level, one falls under involuntary, unconscious brain controls. This three-fold structure remains generally accurate, but, for Myers, it compares with but does not fully explain the co-active layers of the mind. Both middle and lower neural regions would belong to the subliminal self, and the higher to the supraliminal. In current theory the subliminal self conforms to the animal brain.

While epilepsy is the basic model of mental activity, Myers goes on to describe genius as a seizure function. Genius is an on-rush of thought from the subliminal self. Works of genius are regarded as brilliant, because they expand the ordinary range of the mental spectrum into extraordinary radiance. Although genius may split waking consciousness, the intensity of its mental dissociation actually creates a higher integration of the personality. Thus, great works of genius draw us closer to the spiritual world and yet, because of their subliminal origins, they reflect the primitive layers of life.

Myers takes Plato's idea of *eros* (**Symposium**, 192-212) as the prototype of genius. The creative upsurge of genius is an elemental striving of emotion for an everlasting possession of the good. Love as *eros* embodies the basic energy of personal integration that flows more deeply than intellectual thought. *Eros* animates all human faculties in the struggle for the infinite. By stirring up lofty thoughts, *eros* flows "like the swing and libration of the tide-wave across the ocean, which takes no note of billow or of storm" (I, 120). This phrase is quoted in order to show a striking aspect of Myers' writing style, namely, a preference for images of the primal elements, of the sea, fire, and the earth. In other passages, for example, he portrays subliminal activity as "an uprush of the hidden fire" (I, 101); "reverberating tremors [that] rise and fall" and "flood the flats of common consciousness as with the earthquake-wave of an unfathomed sea" (I, 102).

Myers proceeds to describe sleep as the next level of the subliminal self. Sleep is more primitive yet more adaptable than waking consciousness. At the intersection between sleep and waking, nightmares, hypnagogic and hypnopompic images are experienced. Hypnagogic images are those of sight and sound, "faces in the dark," that appear with the coming of sleep; and hypnopompic are those dream-figures that persist into waking consciousness after sleep has ended (I, 125). Hypnopompic figures are shock-forms that evoke pleasure or even ecstasy, as they linger in the mind as afterimages.

Amid the sleep cycle, the dreaming self is independent, having its own faculties and wide-ranging powers, including telepathy, clairvoyance, and transcendent ecstasy. These powers do not evolve through natural selection but emerge from the spiritual capacity inherent in the subliminal self. The dreaming self may be invaded by the spirits of living or dead persons, often accompanied by knowledge of the exact time of death, particularly that of relatives or friends.

The next level of the subliminal self is that of hypnotism or self-suggestion. Cases of spiritual healing are examples of hypnotism, in which the subliminal self generates a rejuvenating energy through suggestion. The subliminal self has a knowledge of the organism, which is deeper than that of waking consciousness and may be activated in times of healing. Rejuvenation occurs in trance states, because the conscious functions of will and attention are inhibited. Healing manifests the profound adaptive power of life itself.

A variation of hypnotic trance is that of a secondary personality, as manifest in possession. Under trance the psyche can change or leave and return to the body, particularly in times of danger or death. The psyche is the same as the spirit or personality, and Myers believes it can withdraw permanently from the body, as exemplified in biological death, but nevertheless retain a relationship with the subliminal self (I, 218). Returning to primal metaphors, Myers explains that personal life is a force, erupting as a "fresh draft" from the cosmic sea of energy.

Myers moves to a conclusion of his first volume with a discussion of sensory automatisms, which are colorful and forceful, visual images that erupt from the subliminal self and penetrate waking consciousness. Some examples are visions, memory-images, creative forms, afterimages, and "the scarlet fire of the epileptic" seizure (I, 228). Despite the analogy with epilepsy, sensory automatisms are not abnormal but are commonly found in persons of sound mental health.

These imaginal forms may be externalized into visions outside the body. Projections of sensory automatisms take place particularly in times of grief, death, or basic change. This ability to transfer imagery outside includes action at a distance, which Myers names "travelling clairvoyance." He illustrates this with the case (666C) of a man sailing on board a ship in the Atlantic Ocean for nine days (I, 682). One night he falls asleep and dreams vividly of his wife, who is actually back home in Connecticut. In the morning his roommate says he also saw the image of the man's wife, during the night. The wife had heard of the storm at sea through the news and, becoming afraid, projected herself across the sea into the ship's room. To account for the projection Myers posits an intermediate concept of psychic space, that is dream-like, independent of matter and having its own extensive continuum (I, 231). This psychic space lies between individual minds and the ultimate cosmic unity of mind. In contemporary thought this is the same as quantum inseparability.

With this notion Myers raises the possibility of communicating after death. Myers and his colleagues had documented many cases of the living having visions of the dead, but he theorized that the spirit of the deceased externalizes itself into a visual form and modifies a portion of space. The spiritual being is psychic, volitional, but without movement. There is no sender-receiver relationship. Rather, the spirit of the deceased breaks through, usually in a dream or vision, to whomever is receptive. Readiness for the psychic breakthrough requires some form of dissociation, as in sleep, for example.

Myers develops a technical concept for this phenomenon, taking over the Greek term *psychorrago*, which means "to let the soul break loose" (I, 264). From this word he constructs the notion of psychorrhagy. Thus, visions of the dead are psychorrhagic in the sense that the spirit of the deceased wills to penetrate the intermediate realm of dream-like space. Such visions may be seen by one person or by several. Whether individual or collective, however, the context of the vision is the subliminal self.

Going on to volume two, Myers continues the same theme but adds more detail. Visions of the dead are called phantasms and are defined as a "manifestation of persistent personal energy," that is, a residue of one's personality when alive (II, 4). The residue is an afterimage, to which Myers attaches the adjective veridical. By veridical afterimage Myers means a real but nonmaterial form, left over after one's death. It is carried by telepathy from the deceased being to the living person, who encounters it unconsciously through a nonpathological dissociation of consciousness. Veridical afterimages seem to erupt like waves from the depths of the subliminal self.

Myers generalizes on how the images act with respect to death. At the onset of the dying process, the subliminal self sends out signals of the impending death. One's awareness of the death becomes clearer and more acute, sometimes involving clairvoyance of the future, for example, seeing deaths of other persons. At the same time, telepathy radiates with friends and relatives, who get premonitions, dreams of the forthcoming death, be compelled to visit the dying person, or have crises of their own. These phenomena obey two distinct processes described in the following two paragraphs.

First, when dying is by disease, psychic activity builds up quickly about one week before death. Shortly after death, it decreases rapidly and gradually slows down until stopping at one year. After the first year, psychic activity may be sporadic or cease altogether. The rapid build up and gradual slow down may be imagined as a wave-like process (II, 14).

Second, when death is unexpected or traumatic, telepathy is suddenly discharged. A current of psychic energy radiates outward from the corpse or death site. The energy may take shape as a field, a spiritual presence, image, or recollection. Whatever form it takes, the energy may linger in one place for many years or be picked up telepathically by the subliminal self of the survivors in visual or aural forms. The radiant fields may even split into specific vibratory forms called hauntings. Suicides and homicides are some examples of shock deaths that release hauntings.

These two conceptual patterns are expressed again in metaphors from the sea. When suggesting that intense concentration may enable hauntings to become manifest to us, he says that in "the boundless ocean of mind innumerable currents and tides shift with the shifting emotion of each several soul" (II, 69). The imagery means that death-induced telepathic exchanges reflect fundamental reality.

From this subject Myers moves to that of motor automatisms, defined as behavioral patterns performed automatically, without will or full self-consciousness, and instigated unconsciously by a secondary self. These too are compared to epilepsy in which a seizure may initiate totally automatic action without any awareness or recollection. However, Myers describes motor automatisms as normal and constructive but not pathological. Automatic writing, possession, and trance mediumship are examples.

To differentiate normal from abnormal motor automatisms Myers advances a thesis, which is crucial to his position: "It may be expected that supernormal vital phenomena will manifest themselves as far as possible through the same channels as abnormal or morbid vital phenomena, when the same centres or the same synergies are involved" (II, 84).

He argues, further, that if a secondary self were to become manifest physiologically, "it seems possible that its readiest *path of externalization*—its readiest outlet of visible action,—may often lie along some track which has already shown to be a line of low resistance by the disintegrating processes of disease." The disease which concerns Myers most is epilepsy; and, therefore, the splitting induced by seizures opens up pathways to the highest level of creative or religious experience. The role played by epilepsy in Myers' life and thought will be explored in chapters one and two.

Automatic writing exemplifies a motor automatism, which combines telepathy with a psychorrhagic invasion of a living person by the spirit of a deceased being. Automatic writing reflects the subliminal self metaphorically, as "profound ocean-currents bear to waves and winds on the surface of the sea" (II, 119). However, manifestation of secondary personalities, in automatic writing, must work through the limitations of the sensory-muscular systems of the living person. Consequently, subliminal messages tend to be simple and repetitive or even projections of one's own unconscious fantasies.

Possession is another example of a motor automatism, and it is related to automatic writing. With possession a conscious person is taken over by a controlling spirit and its own identity or memory. Normally, possession blocks telepathy, although it might break through occasionally. To illustrate possession Myers examines the case of Lenore Piper, a well-known trance medium of Boston. In 1887 she began to fall into trance states, having "a good deal of respiratory disturbance and muscular twitching" (II, 251). A contemporary classics scholar reports that Mrs. Piper suffered epileptic convulsions and symptoms, including the grinding of teeth (Dodds 1971, 228). She would lapse into total unconsciousness, fall forward, and had to be supported. These brief biographical facts illustrate Myers' thesis that epileptic seizures open up channels through which supernormal phenomena flow. After examining Mrs. Piper's mediumship critically, Myers concluded that the spirit of deceased beings retained earthly memories and loves and that they communicated these to the living through trance mediumship (II, 256-257).

Finally, the most profound expression of the subliminal self is ecstasy and as a correlate of trance, it is essentially a religious experience. Ecstasy culminates the spectrum of subliminal activities, beginning with the mental dissociation. Viewed as a whole, the psychic continuum of the subliminal self leads to the knowledge of God through symbolization. Since ecstasy grows out of the extended subliminal self, it is essentially an experience of participation in an exalted transcendent domain. This participation discloses an incandescent unity of life and love, joy and wisdom, and it is most clearly expressed in the symbolism of the distant shore.

From this fundamental insight, Myers draws three specific theological principles. First, love does not die but is stronger than death and deepens as it evolves. Love represents the infinite striving of the self for the realm of spirit, a striving that survives biological death. Love is the exaltation of the law of telepathy (II, 282). Among the religions of the world, Christianity provides a revelation that culminates the telepathic law of the universe. Christianity acknowledges the existence of discarnate beings who love and care for the living. Human life is capable of surviving biological death because of its dual origins: descent from maternal and paternal ancestors and descent from planetary and cosmic heredities.

Second, knowledge of a transcendent, post-mortem world projects no evidence of evil. Messages from the dead, as disclosed through dreams, vision, or trance mediumship speak of neither hell nor torment. Consequently, evil is understood as a purely finite experience traceable to the tragic defects of the human will.

Third, Myers discovered no support for a rigid, cosmic determinism. In some of his case studies, people who acquire subliminal knowledge were able to act so as to avoid danger or death (II, 272). This ability indicates that telepathic law operates according to probabilities and tendencies rather than by fixed action patterns. Dreams and visions of the dead that convey knowledge of earthly affairs reveal a sense of will among the deceased. Such post-mortem communication presupposes the intensity of understanding gained before death.

Ecstatic glimpses of telepathic law disclose the universe to be a vast plenitude of energy, whose mysteries are also the origins of the subliminal self. Though enveloped in mystery, the living are illumined by messages from the dead. For dying is like sailing into an uncharted sea, whose terrors are a revelation of a homecoming. The dying behold a procession of ancestors, or fore-bearers of many generations, moving toward that distant shore, "up through the light of the seas by the moon's long silvering ray" (II, 277).

III. DEATH AND THE SUBLIMINAL SELF

Frederic Myers' theory of the subliminal self contains two original and far-reaching contributions to a psychology of death. One is the concept of telepathy, and the other is that of the veridical afterimage. Telepathy is activated in a wave-like process, either one week before a natural death or suddenly with a shock death, and radiated as a veridical afterimage at the moment of death. The veridical afterimage gradually depletes in its intensity throughout the first year after the death. Implied in this radiant cycle is the fact that every act and thought are preserved subliminally and released in afterimages. Myers compares the radiant shock of death to the death of a star. The dead are like stars that perished eons ago, leaving radiant traces in the night sky.

To illustrate how the subliminal self informs various death experiences, selected case studies from Myers' two volumes are presented below. The subliminal self is activated in dissociative states that relate to epileptic seizures. In some dangerous situations healing energies also radiate subliminally. For example, in case 409B a woman suffers an attack of acute bronchitis, which she fears to be life-threatening. She falls asleep and her sister, who had been dead for more than twenty years,

came to my bedside, and said. "Do not worry about your
health, we have come to cure you; there is much yet for you to
do in the world." Then she vanished, and my brain seemed to
be electrified as if by a shock from a battery, only it was not
painful, but delicious. The shock spread downwards, and over
the chest and lungs it was very strong. From here it extended to
the extremities, where it appeared like a delightful glow. I
awoke almost immediately and found myself well (I, 370).

Two salient points may be drawn from this case. One is that the
telepathic exchange is between two siblings, and the other is that the
radiant shock conforms to the epileptic aura, a glow spreading through
the limbs, which will be discussed in chapter one.

Myers presents several cases in which dreams coincide with the
deaths of family members at distant places. In section 428D a man has
a dream in which an old lady appears, stands, and gazes at him for 20
minutes, neither speaking nor moving. The man does not recognize her,
with her white hair, dark eyebrows, and penetrating eyes. His aunt
comes into the room and says: "John don't you know who this is?" The
woman in the dream is actually the dreamer's grandmother, whose death
on a distant island coincides with the actual dreaming (I, 419). This case
suggests that the knowledge of the death occurs in the subliminal self,
and the dreamwork brings this knowledge into the consciousness of the
dreamer.

Similarly in another case a woman sees "her *headless* brother
standing at the foot of the bed with his head lying on a coffin by his
side" (I, 425). She awakens, then falls asleep and has the same dream
again. For several days the woman grieves for the headless condition of
her brother portrayed in the dream. Some time later, she learns that her
brother, a soldier in Asia, had been decapitated about the time of her
dream.

With terminal illness, telepathy builds up about one week before the
death. Hence, in case 714A a dying man appears in a vision to his
daughter, shortly before his death. She awoke

seeing a bright light in my bedroom—the whole room was
flooded with a radiance quite indescribable—and my father was
standing by my bedside, an etherealized semi-transparent figure,
but yet his voice and his aspect were normal. His voice seemed

a far-off sound, and yet it was his same voice as in life. All he said was, "Take care of mother." He then disappeared, floating in the air, as it were, and the light also vanished (II, 323).

With an unexpected shock death, the radiant telepathy may vibrate in one location, often for many years. Such focused telepathic fields seem to have split-off from the death. In volume two, section 733B, Myers portrays a man and two sisters who are vacationing in a country house owned by friends. One day the elder sister discovers an old woman in bed "with her clothes on and lying with her head towards the window." She calls her sister and brother to enter the room, but when she points to the bed, they see nothing. Hence, the elder sister sees an image of the old woman. She speaks with a neighbor and learns that the previous owner had falsely accused his wife of drinking all of his whiskey. He had become enraged and beaten her to death. Terrified by what he had done, he concealed the murder by telling the neighbor that his wife had suffered a terminal illness. Even though the wife's body had been buried, a visual image of her preterminal state lingered on the bed (II, 360-361).

In a related case (745B) a woman narrates a sighting she had one night about 11 o'clock. She hears someone moaning outside her bedroom window. She raised the window shade and, looking out, "There on the grass was a beautiful young girl in a kneeling posture before a soldier, in a general's uniform, sobbing, and clasping her hands together, entreating for pardon; but alas! he only waved her away from him" (II, 383). The woman runs down the stairs and goes through the outside door to the lawn. Arriving outside, she sees nothing.

After investigating the situation, she learns that the daughter of the previous owner of the house had borne an illegitimate child. Failing to be accepted by her family, she died in grief. The woman also states that the girl and soldier were near relatives and that the soldier had some connection with her husband.

Commenting on this case, Myers admits that he is uncertain as to what extent the deceased is still participating in the post-mortem phantasm (II, 384). Myers' uncertainty presupposes his argument that visions derive from the veridical afterimage. That is, they are instigated by the deceased. However, this case and the one cited above raise the possibility that moral values might be implicated in the veridical afterimage, namely, that the failure to gain forgiveness in a family relationship might be implicated. This possibility needs to be explored by more recent psychologies in subsequent chapters.

A final illustration deals with the near-death experience, something known in the nineteenth century but not extensively examined. In section 713A of the second volume Myers suggests "that we might learn much were we to question dying persons, on their awakening from some comatose condition, as to their memory of any dream or vision during that state" (II, 315). To encourage this practice he cites an 1889 case of a physician who, suffering typhoid fever, sinks into unconsciousness, and loses all pulse and circulation for about four hours. The following paragraph summarizes this case.

Witnesses perceive the doctor to be dead, so they begin funeral preparations. Meanwhile, the "clinically dead" man realizes the essential nature of his personality, and he sees his lifeless body. His ego is rocked back and forth, as it breaks away from the body and floats up and away from it. His mind is alive and intact. He sees people, but they are in an undifferentiated form. He also discovers a cord, through which he is still using his eyes to see. He sees the sky, a mountain, a forest, and a river. Before him stretches a road and, in the distance, large rocks are standing on it as a barrier. Suddenly, fire strikes from the clouds that form a large tent, which revolves on its axis in the sky. Out of the fire, clouds, and tent a spiritual presence appears, saying that this is "the road to the eternal world," and that the rocks are the boundary line between the two worlds. He moves toward the rocks but is stopped by a black cloud, when he awakens.

Myers also quotes a report (663A) in which the same physician had had a clairvoyant episode in 1878, eleven years before his near-death experience. He had a vision of a log house, in which a man killed himself by shooting a rifle into his mouth.

IV. CRITIQUE OF THE SUBLIMINAL SELF

In order to develop constructively Myers' original insights, it is appropriate to consult a critical reaction by one of his contemporaries. He was a close personal friend as well as professional colleague of William James, the distinguished American psychologist. James evaluated Myers' theory of the subliminal self in a memorial address and a book review. These along with James' papers on psychic studies have been published by Gardner Murphy and Robert Ballou (1960). This collection contains a sensitive profile of Myers as a student of death and who suffered Bright's Disease of the kidney which would end his life at age 58,

> Brought up on literature and sentiment, something of a courtier, passionate, disdainful, and impatient naturally, he was made over again from the day when he took up psychical research seriously. He became learned in science, circumspect, democratic in sympathy, endlessly patient, and above all, happy. The fortitude of his last hours touched the heroic, so completely were the atrocious sufferings of his body cast into insignificance by his interest in the cause he lived for. When a man's pursuit gradually makes his face shine and grow handsome, you may be sure it is a worthy one (319-320).

James explains that Myers pioneered in developing a systematic method for psychology, whereby he could coordinate a vast amount of data within a general scheme (217). Myers assembled dissimilar data in series and connected the extremes with intermediary concepts. The theory of the subliminal self is so breath-taking and epochal, because it integrates previously marginal experiences such as seizures, dreams, visions, and ecstatic possession. The latter are normally not unified in theoretical knowledge and likely to be dismissed as superstitious or absurd.

However, by coordinating a large array of seemingly strange phenomena, Myers has developed an original conception of mental evolution, using biological analogies. For James the key to Myers' theory is his contention that consciousness has no essential unity, but is derivative from a wider mental field and useful only as a means of environmental adjustment. Consciousness emerges from biological evolution, but it can dissolve in epilepsy, dreams, and trance. Ironically, the dissolution of consciousness yields a higher mental integration.

More critically, James concedes that the subliminal region exists but does not know whether it pervades all persons or pertains only to a gifted few (228). He believes that the relationships between the subliminal self and the ultimate cosmic unity of mind are vague and ill-defined. James even questions whether Myers' cosmic dimension is truly ultimate or simply a series of subliminal selves (231). Although Myers' work is a masterpiece, a vision of the highest intellectual order, it invites the following criticisms: (1) some of Myers' facts need more verification; (2) some of the claims of universality are not warranted; and (3) the theory is a generalization from exceptional cases (235).

Behind these criticisms lurk a fundamental issue which troubles James. He cannot come to terms with Myers' claim cited above, "that supernormal vital phenomena will manifest themselves as far as possible through the same channels as abnormal or morbid vital phenomena" (237). Essentially, James cannot understand how epilepsy reveals a transcendent spiritual realm.

Nevertheless, toward the end of his life, James arrived at conclusions basically the same as Myers'. Mystical experience, the ground of all religion, is a "possession of an extended subliminal self" (265). Messages erupt from it, in times of mental dissociation, and produce dreams, trance, and so forth. The threshold of the mind is lowered, so that transcendent knowledge may filter through the dissociated self. This assumes that the brain has a transmissive function and that it is open and not closed.

James even speaks with the same imagery as does Myers. The conscious personality is like an island in a cosmic sea. The subliminal self is like the ocean, whose waves beat upon the shores of the conscious ego as volcanic eruptions. Memories of our earthly existence are stored unconsciously in the subliminal self, and, after death, they erupt in dreams, visions, and trance mediumship. Thus, the dialogue between James and Myers bequeathed to the twentieth century the problems of epilepsy, death, and selfhood.

CHAPTER ONE:
EPILEPSY AND THE OTHER WORLD

I. DR. Z. AND HIS BROTHER

Frederic Myers' theory of the subliminal self rests upon the paradoxical interaction of the abnormal and the supernormal. His model of the abnormal is epilepsy, and he contends that epileptic seizures open up the psyche to transcendent states. When viewed historically, Myers' conception of epilepsy reflects a pivotal, transitional phase in modern medicine. Known in Greek antiquity as the "sacred disease," in the Christian era epilepsy became "the falling sickness" and was frequently diagnosed as the effect of possession. However, beginning with the nineteenth century psychiatry made systematic observations of epileptics and formulated basic personality traits of the disease. This development was facilitated by the founding of asylums and epileptic wards in general hospitals in France, Germany, and England. These asylum doctors discovered a unique character behind the symptoms, created a new terminology, and developed statistical studies (Temkin 1971, 257).

The asylum doctors clarified types of seizures that remain well known. Grand mal seizure meant a total bodily convulsion with loss of consciousness. Petit mal seizures consisted of a range of attacks considered less severe. Absence entailed a temporary loss of consciousness without convulsions. The *furor epilepticus* comprised a premonition, noise in the head, threatening dreams, loss of consciousness, falling, and release of homicidal rage.

Two French physicians, Benedict Morel and Jules Falret, found anger and irritability to be basic characteristics of the epileptic. Any trivial incident could trigger epileptoid anger, lasting one or two hours and even repeating during the day. Anger could appear just before or after a seizure; or it could exist independently and be discharged spontaneously in violent actions. The epileptic seizure would be expressed in an attack, fall, or a dizzy spell, i.e. vertigo. On the other hand the condition could be hidden in specific behavior without convulsions, in a state known as masked epilepsy (*épilepsie larvée*).

In the same era, German psychiatrists produced the concept of psychic equivalents, stating that an epileptic could have symptoms that were independent of but equal to seizures. As in Myers' theory, one of the psychic equivalents of epilepsy was the experience of a transcendent world in a deep state of trance. Within the seizure one has a vision, which could be remembered after the convulsion. The following letter, written by an epileptic patient to his wife, illustrates this psychic equivalent:

> I then thought that I was caught up by the hair of my head, and brought through the air to a beautiful country, which was surrounded by beautiful green grass parks, and those parks were full of young lambs,...I then asked the person supposed to be in my company, where was God. His reply was in Heaven. I then said this was Heaven. He then said that this was only a kitchen to Heaven, and none can enter into Heaven but those that are pure and perfect. He, the visionary man, said that this was the place that saints were made perfect in. He then told me the number that had entered since our Savior went there (cited in Temkin 1971, 372).

Such epileptic patients sincerely believed that they were in heaven, had left their bodies, visited the divine region, and returned to their bodies. They ascribed heavenly status to themselves and to their doctors. Having recalled their visions proves that not all awareness was lost, while they were unconscious. The trance consisted of a twilight state, in which the threshold of consciousness was lowered but not entirely extinguished, Although epileptic attacks might have been followed by phases of confusion or depression, patients remained pleasant, amiable, and gentle.

When Myers was formulating his position, during the latter third of nineteenth century, neurology emerged to compete with psychiatry and to establish medical dominance. The neurological study of epilepsy was founded by the British physician John Hughlings Jackson. In the 1860s Jackson observed epileptic fits occurring on one side of the body, having no loss of consciousness, but yet exhibiting impaired sight, speech defects, and an aura of a foul smell at the onset of the attack. Jackson interpreted this unilateral seizure as a sudden local discharge of grey matter in the brain. Avoiding broad generalizations, he argued that the different kinds of attacks conform to the evolutionary hierarchy of the brain. Epilepsy proper, involving loss of consciousness, originates in the highest brain centers, but localized seizures, called epileptiform attacks derive from the middle brain region. Jackson recognized a third, miscellaneous class of fits, as found in breathing disturbances or injuries, that pertain to the lower level of the brain. He theorized that epilepsy reversed the order of evolution through a descending process of mental dissolution, i.e. from the higher level to the lowest.

So-called Jacksonian epilepsy means that specific types of seizures correlate directly with organic disease in the brain. Brain disease is purely physiological. Psychological symptoms are useful only as signs that point to particular disturbances in the brain. For Jackson the brain embraces a configuration of movements, which is essentially separate from but parallel to moral or emotional symptoms. While fear may precede an attack, the fundamental cause is a discharging lesion in the movements of the brain.

The actual birth of neurology took place in London on January 10, 1894, when one of Jackson's epileptic patients died. Jackson asked to be present at the autopsy of this patient, known in medical history as Dr. Z.. Jackson persuaded his colleague Walter Colman, who conducted the autopsy, to search "the taste region of Ferrier on each half of the brain very carefully;" and they found "a very small focus of softening in that region (in the uncinate gyrus) of the left half of the brain" (Jackson 1931, 461). The name Ferrier was that of David Ferrier, who studied experimentally the conductive fibers to the brain, which supported Jackson's observation of local convulsions induced by the discharge of grey matter. The autopsy discovered the lesion in the left temporal lobe of the brain. Jackson's account of this autopsy in his published papers became the neurological paradigm of temporal lobe epilepsy in the twentieth century.

Jackson founded neurology as a mechanistic and physiological science. He maintained a strict psycho-physical dualism, sharply separating the fields of psychology and medicine, and restricting the latter to physiology. Whereas the asylum doctors had studied types of convulsions and states of consciousness, Jackson focused on the morbid condition of brain cells. For Jackson the greater the discharge of grey matter in the brain, then the more severe would be the seizure. Study of the biography of the patient, which the asylum doctors had conducted, was neglected.

After Jackson's pioneering work, neurology expanded and, by the mid-twentieth century, dominated the understanding of epilepsy. The triumph of neurology was aided by the introduction of the EEG in 1929, making possible more precise readings of brain activities. For example, the concept of psychomotor epilepsy replaced Jackson's "uncinate group of epileptic fits," and its origins in the temporolimbic region in the brain was documented (Blumer 1984, 37). Meanwhile, the identity of Dr. Z. remained unknown, and he passed into historical oblivion. Because Jackson ignored the person behind the symptoms, his successors failed to ask a simple question: Who was Dr. Z.?

Nearly 100 years after the famous autopsy, David Taylor and Susan Marsh identified Dr. Z. as Arthur T. Myers (1980). Born in 1851 Arthur Myers was the youngest son of Rev. Frederic Myers, a priest in the Church of England. The father also died in 1851, at the age of 40, only a few months after Arthur was born. Arthur was the youngest brother of Ernest Myers and of Frederic W. H. Myers—theorist of the subliminal self. Is this family relationship the reason why Frederic Myers made epilepsy the paradigm of the subliminal self?

Arthur Myers' obituary was published in the **British Medical Journal** on January 27, 1894 and reprinted by Taylor and Marsh (1980, 760-761). A few biographical facts reveal the decedent's epileptic personality. Myers was educated at Cheltenham and Trinity College, Cambridge. He received his medical degree in 1881 and in 1893 became a Fellow in the College of Physicians. He practiced at St. George's Hospital and Belgrave Hospital for Children, where his work was characterized by "patience, minuteness, and fidelity." Myers published papers in leading journals and displayed an interest in psychological problems and psychic research. He was an outstanding athlete, winning several prizes in racketball and tennis. Despite his great athletic prowess,

> destiny thought fit to inflict upon him that terrible and inscrutable nervous malady which occasionally harassed him in

early youth, and of late years advanced with relentless tread, baffling the most devoted medical skill and ultimately involving a fine intellect in ruin and confusion.

[He] was of a singularly kind and amiable disposition, given much to acts of hospitality and goodness to others. The slight brusqueness of his address, sometimes remarked by his juniors, was largely due to his infirmity....His history is tinged with a touch of melancholy,...for he has shown us the example of a brave man struggling against an unhappy fate (760).

Arthur Myers was a life-long bachelor who died at 42. Taylor and Marsh contend convincingly that Myers' death was a suicide committed by an overdose of chloral hydrate (758, 763-764). The death was not judged legally to be a suicide, but they argue from the cumulative and lethal effects of asphyxia, coma, epilepsy, Bright's Disease of the kidneys, and narcotic medications.

The biography is significant, further, because it yields the sources of some of Jackson's basic concepts. Jackson's publications contain verbatim accounts by Arthur Myers of his own seizure experiences. One example, reported by Jackson in July 1888, is as follows:

I first noticed symptoms which I subsequently learnt to describe as *petit-mal* when living at one of our universities, 1871. I was in very good general health, and knew of no temporary disturbing causes. I was waiting at the foot of a College staircase, in the open air, for a friend who was coming down to join me. I was carelessly looking round me, watching people passing, etc., when my attention was suddenly absorbed in my own mental state, of which I know no more than that it seemed to me to be a vivid and unexpected "recollection"—of what, I do not know. My friend found me a minute or two later, leaning my back against the wall, looking rather pale, and feeling puzzled and stupid for the moment (Jackson 1931, 400).

More attacks came in the next two years. Often at night he would awaken "with an impression that I had succeeded in recollecting something that I wanted to recollect" but then had forgotten it by morning. On awakening he would have soreness at the edge of the tongue, a feeling of having been bitten, and saliva on the pillow.

Generalizing on his seizures, Myers states that the sense of recollection was central, namely, "realizing that what is occupying the attention is what had occupied it before, and indeed has been familiar, but has been for a time forgotten, and now is recovered...." (Jackson 1931, 401) This statement actually anticipates Sigmund Freud's definition of the unconscious, which will be discussed in chapter two. Myers admits that his normal memory is poor but "in the abnormal states the recollection is much more instantaneous, much more absorbing, more vivid, and for the moment more satisfactory, as filling up a void which I imagine at the time I had previously in vain sought to fill." The recollections always begin "by another person's voice, or by my own verbalised thought." Then the return to normal consciousness is not a rush but a gradual process. Return to consciousness is marked by a flush in the skin and face, quickened heart beat, and increased urinary output.

During seizure, Myers becomes pale and has an empty look in the eyes, assenting to anyone's remarks. Saying yes includes a smacking of the tongue or a tasting movement of the lower jaw. After a *petit-mal* attack, he neither hallucinates nor loses balance. Myers recalls running across a Swiss glacier in 1878, when an aura befell him:

> I had insufficient control to stop myself and felt no fear, but only a slight interest in what would happen. I went through the familiar sensations of *petit-mal* with such attention as I had to give concentrated on them, and not on the ice, and after a few minutes regained my normal condition without any injury. I looked back with surprise at the long slope of broken ice I had run over unhurt, picking my way, I know not how, over ground that would normally have been difficult to me (Jackson 1931, 403).

Myers began to suffer grand mal seizures after 1874, and normally they recurred at intervals of 18 months. When recovering from pneumonia in 1876, he had seven or eight attacks within a two month span. An aura of recollection followed his grand mal convulsions, but it lacked the clarity of those after the petit mal. With the grand mal neither an epileptic cry was heard nor muscular spasms observed. Nevertheless, he felt tired and sore with bodily bruises.

Myers recalls several episodes, when a seizure would come and yet, despite the absence of memory and consciousness, he could still function physically and purposefully. In one situation, he saw a young male patient, who complained of lung problems. Myers told the young man to undress and lie down on the couch, so as to be examined.

> I thought he looked ill, but have no recollection of any intention to recommend him to take to his bed at once, or of any diagnosis. Whilst he was undressing I felt the onset of a *petit-mal*. I remember taking out my stethoscope and turning away a little to avoid conversation. The next thing I recollect is that I was sitting at a writing-table in the same room, speaking to another person, and as my consciousness became more complete, recollected my patient, but saw he was not in the room (Jackson 1931, 404-405).

One hour later, Myers observed the patient in bed and read, in the patient's chart, his diagnosis of pneumonia. He concluded that both his conscious and his unremembered diagnoses were, in fact, the same.

Jackson also reports that occasionally there were post-paroxysmal, purposive "actions by Z during 'unconsciousness,' of a kind which in a man fully himself would be criminal, and must have led to very serious consequences had not fortunately, his condition been known. What he did was overlooked by those concerned" (1931, 460). Myers' "criminal" actions remain unknown, but in light of the findings by the asylum doctors, violent or indiscreet sexual deeds are possibilities. In the same context, Jackson asserts that Dr. Z. suffered anxiety. "It was not a fear of the fit; the dread came first, and then the fit, or rather the rest of the fit."

Myers' own introspective statements gave rise directly to the distinctive concepts of Jacksonian epilepsy: "dreamy state," "intellectual aura," *deja vu*, and familiar yet strange premonitions. When produced under seizure, Myers' writings exhibit normal grammatical structure, but the words are written in a round-about, confusing manner. Otherwise, his writings are clear, coherent, and compact. When combining these biographical facts with additional traits known to the asylum doctors, the classical psychiatric profile of epilepsy emerges. Myers was charitable and pleasant, his work habits precise and dutiful; and yet he was sad, melancholy, and irritable (Blumer 1984, 25). He chose not to marry, a fact implying a lack of sexual arousal or interest. Myers was also concerned with the supernatural world and psychic ability, by virtue of his relationship with his brother Frederic (Taylor and Marsh (1980, 761). Though open to psychic experiences of the other world, he retained a scientific scepticism. His critical bent and medical knowledge aided his brother in the conceptualization of the subliminal self. In the preface of his first volume, Frederic acknowledges his brother's help. "My thanks are due also to another colleague who has passed away, my brother, Dr. A. T. Myers, F.R.C.P., who helped me for many years in all medical points arising in the work" (1903/1954, I ix).

Finally, my intent in this chapter is to correlate the epilepsy of Arthur Myers with the vision of the other world in the intellectual work of his brother Frederic. Since Frederic Myers regarded epilepsy as the paradigm of abnormal, dissociated consciousness, surely this belief comes from his family relationship. Further, it is my intent to argue, more fully in the next chapter, that (1) the theory of the subliminal self is a sublimation of threshold epilepsy and that (2) Frederic Myers' selection of eruptive images (e.g. fire, ocean waves, and earthquakes) is driven unconsciously by an inherited familial tendency. It is not my intent to account for all the functions of the subliminal self but to integrate its epileptoid character with specific death experiences in order to achieve a symbolic framework, useful to clinical work and theological reflection.

Correlating Arthur Myers' disease with his brother's theoretical vision presupposes the validity of psychiatric findings, established before the introduction of the EEG and anticonvulsant medications. As stated above, neurology has dominated the study of epilepsy in the twentieth century. Neurology has converged with pharmacology and provided successful treatment for epileptic patients. They can live normal lives without the crippling effects or social stigma of the seizures. Medical success has led to the common assumption that epilepsy is only a brain disorder, having no psychiatric complications. Epilepsy is no longer perceived as the falling sickness.

However, a closer look at epilepsy will reveal that although they be denied and medically treated, the psychiatric aspects of the falling sickness do not disappear (Blumer and Benson 1982). The major convulsions may be controlled, but the personality traits discovered by the asylum doctors remain in place. The only change is that the epileptoid character has become more subtle, muted, and likely to be overlooked (Blumer, et. al. 1988, 118-121). An example of this situation will be presented in the last section of this chapter.

When viewed historically, the separation of neurology and psychiatry rests upon two philosophical assumptions, flowing from Jackson's analysis of the Dr. Z. autopsy. Neurology concentrated on the physical brain cells as the object of scientific investigation, while splitting off the subjective personality and family relationships. By focusing on the brain as object, neurologists presume reality to be physical and, therefore, prefer monistic, epiphenomenal, and dualistic interpretations. Consequently, behavioral traits in the personality, family, or genealogy lack intrinsic significance. As Jackson said, psychological tendencies are only signs of a neural lesion.

In contrast, my intent is to integrate subject and object, person and family, assuming that reality consists of relatedness. With respect to epilepsy a comprehensive understanding needs the unification of neurology and psychiatry (cf. Szondi 1980, 192-193; Blumer 1984, 52-57). The union of these two disciplines moves the subject of epilepsy beyond the monistic and dualistic assumptions of the age of Jackson. In a unified, medical perspective, personality characteristics are not merely signs but are unconscious channels of transcendent reality.

II. THE DOSTOEVSKY AURA

The fundamental psychiatric profile of epilepsy bears a polarity of pent-up emotion and ethical, religious, and/or psychic experiences of an other world. To understand how this polarity helps shape a psychology of death it is appropriate to consider the experience of Fyodor Dostoevsky. This eminent Russian writer suffered epilepsy nearly his entire life, and his personal life-world, as revealed in his literary characters, was the same as that of Arthur Myers. Furthermore, Dostoevsky's life and work exhibit almost all the phases of the subliminal self: disintegration, genius, sensory automatisms, phantasms of the dead, motor automatisms, and ecstatic trance. By carefully recording his own seizures and reading medical literature, Dostoevsky worked out a precise and detailed understanding of the classical psychomotor or temporal lobe epilepsy. During the last twenty years of his life, 1861-1881, when he wrote his great works with epileptic characters, the French asylum doctors shaped the medical paradigm of epilepsy. Dostoevsky's characters essentially replicated that model.

Dostoevsky's epilepsy appeared between 1846-1848, although epileptiform symptoms in the sense of nervous disorders were present in his childhood. His letters give evidence of epileptic symptoms before they were actually diagnosed. In a letter to his older brother Mikhail, dated February 1, 1846, Dostoevsky admits his fear of a "nervous fever," and in a subsequent letter on July 18, 1849, he complains of a "disorder of the nerves that goes in a *crescendo*. Now and then I have throat spasms like the ones I used to have before" and "I have bad nightmares" (Frank and Goldstein 1987, 37, 45). He also suffered poor appetite, hemorrhoids and diarrhea, heightened sensitivity, long dreams, and occasionally loss of a sense of time.

Other early symptoms included auditory hallucinations, dizziness, and fainting spells, the latter occurring with an aura. At the time, the aura was conceived as a "breeze," since this was the translation of the classical Latin term, which had been introduced by the Roman physician Galen. He identified the aura as a sensation moving through bodily limbs before erupting in a seizure. In Dostoevsky's experience the aura appeared a few seconds or minutes at the onset of the attack. Along with the aura he had premonitory signs, called prodromatas, a few hours or days before the convulsion, including ill-temper, absences, drowsiness, and depression (Rice 1985, 10-11).

Having endured all these symptoms for several years, Dostoevsky consulted a physician, Stephen Yanovsky, for a diagnosis. He would diagnose Dostoevsky correctly in 1847, observe his seizures, and report his psychic interests. Both doctor and novelist developed a close bond, so that their relationship itself took on a psychic quality. Yanovsky lived in Pavlovsk and travelled to St. Petersburg three times a week for his medical practice. He recalls that one

> day a strange urge convinced him of the necessity of returning to the city for an unscheduled visit. In a remote area he accidentally ran into Dostoevsky who had no money to pay a petty debt demanded of him by some military clerk. When the writer saw the doctor, he shouted, "See! See who will save me!" Later Dostoevsky called the incident remarkable and every time he would remember it, he would say, "Well, after that, how could one not believe in premonitions!" (Berry 1981, 44).

In this situation Yanovsky discovered Dostoevsky suffering convulsions, agitation, blood rushing to the head, and arms bleeding. Viewing the episode in terms of Frederic Myers' theory of the subliminal self, we might infer that Yanovsky and Dostoevsky shared a telepathic exchange, triggered by the writer's life-threatening convulsion.

A second situation, witnessed by Yanovsky, came about one year later in the early morning hours of May 29, 1848:

> After two I heard extremely raucous heavy gasps, and when I went into F. M.'s room with a lighted candle I saw him lying on his back with eyes open, in convulsions, with foam at his mouth and his tongue sticking out. Here for the first time I saw the illness in an extreme degree (cited in Rice 1985, 11).

Yanovsky's observation illustrates Dostoevsky's life-long pattern of undergoing convulsions during sleep which may have persisted undetected throughout his childhood. After nocturnal attacks, he would awaken in pain, bleeding, bruised, and aching. In the nineteenth century it was known that epilepsy could simulate death, and Dostoevsky feared being mistaken for dead and buried alive.

The relationship between death and epilepsy was clarified, further, by Dostoevsky's mock execution. On April 23, 1849, he was arrested for participating in revolutionary circles and condemned to death by a firing squad. Standing on the scaffold, waiting to be shot, he felt a "mystic terror," just like that in his epileptic seizures (Frank 1983, 55). As narrated in **The Idiot** he recalled having only five minutes to live, and in that brief moment his thinking accelerated with a heightened clarity:

> Not far off there was a church, and the gilt roof was glittering in the bright sunshine. He remembered that he stared very persistently at that roof and the light flashing from it; he could not tear himself away from the light. It seemed to him that those rays were his new nature and that in three minutes he would somehow melt into them (Garnett, trans. 1958, 57).

With the roll of the drum, unexpectedly, Dostoevsky's death sentence was commuted and followed by a four-year prison term in Siberia. Nevertheless, in those few minutes facing the firing squad, he came to know the purification of the end of time and the "eternity of life."

Subsequently, in 1868, when Dostoevsky published **The Idiot**, he included a sketch of the phases of his epilepsy: (1) He would have prodromatas, feeling sick, absent-minded, dreamy, and agitated. These signs would make him sad, oppressed, and mentally dark. Then, one minute before the convulsion, light flashed like lightning in his brain and, suddenly, his vital forces intensified:

> The sense of life, the consciousness of self, were multiplied ten times at these moments which passed like a flash of lightning. His mind and heart were flooded with extraordinary light; all his uneasiness, all his doubts, all his anxieties were relieved at once; they were all merged in a lofty calm, full of serene, harmonious joy and hope (218).

Speaking through his epileptic character Prince Myshkin, Dostoevsky asks: What if the light were a disease? He answers his own questioning by claiming that even if it were abnormal, it would not matter, so long as it is "the acme of harmony and beauty, and gives a feeling, unknown and undivided till then, of completeness, of proportion, of reconciliation, and of ecstatic devotional merging in the highest synthesis of life" (218). Then in the same context he declares that he would gladly sacrifice his entire life for the ecstasy of this aura, when: "There shall be no more time." (219) The latter statement is a quotation of Revelation 10:6, and it means that in the apocalypse clock time (*chronos*) comes to an end.

(2) The light would go out and total darkness would descend with violent convulsions:

> At the moment the face is horribly distorted, especially the eyes. The whole body and the features of the face work with convulsive jerks and contortions. A terrible, indescribable scream that is unlike any thing else breaks from the sufferer. In that scream everything human becomes obliterated (227).

To a by-stander it seems that someone else inside is screaming, and the sight evokes horror and the uncanny.

(3) After the seizure, which takes several days to get over, one feels sadness and depression. Memory and the logical connections of ideas are ruptured. Everything seems strange and uncanny; meanwhile, the body feels heavy. A profound sense of guilt pervades the depression, a feeling that one had committed a crime long ago.

(4) The epileptic is vulnerable to peculiar personality states between the seizures. One wanders aimlessly, unaware of other people, feeling restless, strained, and the need to be alone. During this intermediate phase, one may have a *deja vu*, paranoia, and extreme fear, as well as religious feelings.

From 1861 to 1881, the last twenty years of his life, Dostoevsky recorded 102 seizures. The attacks varied from twice a day to those at intervals of four or five months. Some were preceded by premonitions, others by auras. The fury of the attacks was heightened by throat spasms, which aroused his earlier dread of death, including fears of dying in sleep or of being wrongly pronounced dead and buried alive. The throat spasms also awakened fears of suffocating and choking to death.

Notes written by Dostoevsky between June 16-28, 1870, illustrate Frederic Myers' notion of "phantasms of the dead:"

> At night I saw my brother in a dream, he'd seemingly been resurrected but was living separately from the family. I seemed to be at his place, and somehow I seemed to be not right: loss of consciousness, just like fainting spells. I don't think...I went into some large room nearby to consult a doctor. Brother was seemingly more gentle toward me. I awoke, again fell asleep, and the dream seemed to continue (Cited in Rice 1985, 292).

The brother is Mikhail, who died of liver disease on July 6, 1864. Dostoevsky goes on to describe the second part of the dream:

> I see my father (for a long time I've not dreamt of him). He directs my attention toward my chest, below the right nipple, and said: "All's well with you, but here it is very bad." I looked and it actually seemed that there was some kind of growth below the nipple. Father said: "Your nerves are in disorder." Then at father's there's some kind of family holiday, and his old mother entered, my granny, and all my ancestors. He was happy. From his words I concluded that I was in a very bad way. I showed the other doctor my chest, he said: "Yes, it's right there. You haven't long to live; you are in your final days."

Dostoevsky explains that, after awakening in the morning, he felt a painful, bruised spot on his chest, exactly where his father, a physician, pointed in the dream. He also states that his lungs fill up with liquid, and he has trouble breathing.

Dostoevsky discussed a repetition of this dream in a subsequent letter on April 28, 1871, to his second wife Anna: "I dreamed last night of *my father* and he appeared to me in a terrifying guise, such as he has only appeared to me twice before in my life, both times prophesying a dreadful disaster, and on both occasions the dream came true" (Frank and Goldstein 1987, 353-354). The message conveyed by the dream was accurate, because Dostoevsky suffered progressive pulmonary disease during the last eleven years of his life. The clinical significance of the dream is twofold. It is an authentic precognitive dream, with a familial telepathic exchange, and consistent with the case material used by Frederic Myers for his theory of the subliminal self. It incorporates aspects of the ancestral dream (Szondi 1963, 84) which will be developed further in chapter four.

In the same year of the dream Dostoevsky published **The Possessed** and, speaking through the epileptic Kirillov, clarified the aura further:

There are seconds—they come five or six at a time—when you suddenly feel the presence of the eternal harmony perfectly attained. It's something not earthly—I don't mean in the sense that it's heavenly—but in that sense that man cannot endure it in his earthly aspect. He must be physically changed or die. This feeling is clear and unmistakable; it's as though you apprehend all nature and suddenly say, "Yes, that's right." God, when He created the world, said at the end of each day of creation, "Yes, it's right, it's good." It...it's not being deeply moved, but simply joy. You don't forgive anything because there is no more need of forgiveness. It's not that you love—oh, there's something in it higher than love—what's most awful is that it's terribly clear and such joy. If it lasted more than five seconds, the soul could not endure it and must perish. In those five seconds I live through a lifetime, and I'd give my whole life for them, because they are worth it (Garnett, trans. 1936, 601).

Here Dostoevsky specifies joy as the essence of the aura, and its intensity is metaphysical in the sense of disclosing the whole of Creation. He continues:

I think man ought to give up having children—what's the use of children, what's the use of evolution when the goal has been attained? In the gospel it is written that there will be no child-bearing in the resurrection, but that men will be like the angels of the Lord.

The gospel, to which Dostoevsky refers, is Matthew, stating; "For in the resurrection they neither marry nor are given in marriage, but are like angels in heaven" (22:30). The context is eschatological; joy manifests ultimate reality as revealed in the death experience. The absence of child-bearing complements and does not contradict the joy.

Dostoevsky's lung disease, which was revealed in the dream of his father, deteriorated into pulmonary tuberculosis. His epileptic seizures ceased in 1878, three years before his death on January 28, 1881. The apparent cause of his death was a hemorrhaging of the blood vessels, which filled the lungs (Burke 1969, 687). The vessels had eroded as a result of the progressive tuberculosis. Weakened by an enormous loss of blood, Dostoevsky had a premonition of his coming death. He made a confession and took the Holy Communion (Frank and Goldstein 1987, 515). He remained conscious up to the moment of his death and then passed into the mystery of the eternal.

III. PAROXYSMAL-EPILEPTIFORM PATTERN

In his masterful history of epilepsy Owsei Temkin argues that the Dostoevsky aura was a literary device to shape the story and not a direct expression of the disease (1971, 377). Temkin's position can no longer be maintained; for nearly 100 years after Dostoevsky's death, an Italian research team confirmed the medical existence of the ecstatic aura. The case involved an unmarried, 30 year old male, whose epileptic attacks began at age 13. His seizures came in relaxed or drowsy states, inducing a detachment from the environment, followed by indescribable joy, feeling of total bliss, and without any negative thought or sensation (Cirignotta, et. al., 1980, 709).

The medical confirmation of the aura also raises a question as to whether the basic polarity of epilepsy, i.e. pent-up emotion and ethical, religious, and/or psychic interests, might be more than metaphorical. Temkin wrote his history with the expectation that Jacksonian neurology would eliminate epilepsy altogether (1971, 388). Temkin's hope presumes that Jacksonian etiology, namely, an epileptogenic lesion in the temporolimbic system, would completely explain the falling sickness. However, the neuropsychiatrist Dietrich Blumer challenges the assumption that the complexity of epilepsy can be explained by a simple lesion in the brain. He finds that the basic polarity entails a dynamic tension of polar factors, which are found in varying degrees among healthy people as well (Blumer 1984, 53). Blumer believes a broader genetic factor is necessary to account for both the neurological and psychiatric aspects. His judgment is consistent with the trend in genetics to conceive of multifactorial causation of epilepsy (Lennox 1951), an inheritance in which major genes or polygenes interact with endocrine and exogenous factors, producing thresholds of liability for the disease (Andermann 1980). Blumer appeals to the comprehensive theory of epilepsy, as worked out by his teacher Leopold Szondi.

As early as the 1920s, Szondi began pioneering investigations of neuropsychiatric problems, using extensive pedigree studies and a multi-generational family perspective. For example, by 1931 he determined that neuroses bear multifactorial causation, specifically heredity, the psychobiological constitution of the brain, and midbrain disturbances. This view came out of his pioneering study of stuttering as a global dysfunctional phenomenon rather than as the pathology of a particular organ. In 1932 Szondi demonstrated that stuttering is genetically related to migraines and epilepsy. Between 1932-1935 he established the fact that epilepsy, migraines, and stuttering obey a dimer recessive pattern of inheritance with quantitative variations of multiple alleles (Szondi 1936, 331-333). In European medicine epilepsy, migraines, and stuttering are called the "Szondi Triad."

After showing the hereditary character of neuroses, Szondi went on to demonstrate that they vary with respect to different genetic groups. Some belong to the predominantly schizoform group, others to that of the manic-depressive group. However, epilepsy, migraines, and stuttering represent the paroxysmal group, which is characterized by the "attack" syndrome, namely: (1) an accumulation and release of emotions and (2) inclination to hide one's face (Szondi 1977, 482). The two paroxysmal tendencies of this syndrome are shared by humans and animals.

The human being is a hierarchically-ordered whole system that has evolved with both a high-level mental integration as well as an instinctual drive nature. Such basic wholeness precludes the argument that a single gene or simple brain lesion is the sole determinant of a specific behavior. It is necessary to recognize an intermediate level between simple factors and the whole, in order to unite distinctly human and animal functions. The intermediate level in the human organism contains instinctual drive systems, which are genetically-derived and evolutionarily stable. Instinctual drives belong to the animal brain.

The instinctual drive operating in epilepsy is the paroxysmal pattern. In typical medical usage the term paroxysmal designates, on the one hand, fever or tachycardia and, on the other, convulsions. Here paroxysmal denotes an intensification of energy to a climax, followed by a rest (Szondi 1987, 263). The sequence of rising up and slowing down constitutes a rhythm which unfolds through repetitions. When viewed through a span of time, the rhythmic recurrences display a wave-like undulating process.

Szondi's concept of the paroxysmal pattern resembles, to a certain extent, the biological startle pattern, which is a universal, involuntary reaction to shock and a preparation for danger. In popular thought the startle readies a "fight or flight" reaction. However, the unique feature of Szondi's concept is that the startle intensifies energy which drives against death not only in defense against its threat but as a search for meaning and value. When the intensification of energy informs an epileptic seizure, a volcanic eruption of emotion flows against the danger and becomes transformed into a death-like state (Szondi 1977, 494). As a defense, one is put into the place of death by the release of hostile emotion (*sich-selbst-tot-stellen*). The specific biological mechanism is called the "death-feigning reflex" (*Totstellreflex*).

The paroxysmal pattern may be analyzed in terms of two branches. In the one, the "death-feigning reflex" discharges crude pent-up emotion in the form of epileptic seizures; in the other, the inclination to hide one's face is a reflex involving motor disturbances, blushing and becoming pale, as well as mimicry in the form of hysterical attacks (Szondi 1960, 102). Epilepsy is a defense against the threat of death, hysteria a defense against imaginary danger. Epileptic seizures frequently occur at night and in sleep, hysterical outbursts in daytime and waking consciousness. With EEG measurements it is possible to refine more precisely the differences between epilepsy and hysteria, but clinically they are both convulsive in nature, sharing the "attack" syndrome.

One of Szondi's fundamental insights is that epilepsy, in particular, satisfies certain needs and tendencies, which vary in terms of normality or abnormality, and which possess a polarity. The task is to explain the essential polarity of epilepsy, namely, the discharge of pent-up emotion and ethical, religious, psychic activities. This polarity is exemplified by clinically diagnosed epileptics like Arthur Myers and Dostoevsky and in less extreme modes by persons of similar or related heredity. The paroxysmal pattern of epilepsy may be conceptualized by the following model:

(1) Accumulation of gross affects (e.g. anger, rage, envy, jealousy, hatred, vengeance). This is called the Cain tendency by Szondi, and it accounts for the irritability and anger of the epileptic, as the asylum doctors observed.

(2) Acceleration of affects to a peak, causing convulsion and a lowered threshold of consciousness. One becomes passive, involuntary, seemingly unaware, and capable of committing violence.

(3) Movement toward atonement through love, courage, passion, compassion, desire, and joy. This is called the Abel tendency, and it informs moral action, religious faith, and psychic grasp of a transcendent realm.

This model accounts for the clinically observed cases of classical psychiatry and the introspective statements by epileptics themselves. It pertains to the basic forms of epilepsy as well as to their psychic equivalents, such as all vascular disturbances, allergies, glaucoma, bed-wetting, and severe psychotic psychopathologies (Szondi 1963, 336). Additional equivalents are infantile eclampsia, asthma, left-handedness, and tendencies toward violent death (Szondi 1972, 93, 107).

From the age of the asylum doctors to the present, psychiatry has recognized secondary traits in the epileptic character, which are tendencies toward clinging, tenacious and perseverative behavior toward people and ideas (Szondi 1963, 333). Contemporary psychiatric studies add even more secondary characteristics: round-about writing style; compulsive, verbose speaking or writing; and close attention to details (Bear, et. al. 1984; Himmelhoch 1984). These traits are acknowledged in contemporary neurology, but they are derived from the temporal lobe as transient instabilities that only evoke psychic seizures in the form of anxiety (Persinger 1987, 16, 134). In contrast, Szondi argues that the epileptic personality clings, perseveres, and so forth, not because of anxiety, but in order to control anger, jealousy, or hatred. This presupposes the classical psychiatric insight that hostile emotions are eruptive and volcanic, thereby making anxiety a secondary aspect of seizures.

One of the major discoveries of contemporary psychiatry is the fact that the epileptic lacks sexual activity, arousal, or interest, whether male or female, young or old. This fact was established in a pioneering study conducted by Henri Gastaut and Henri Collomb (1954). Hyposexuality is the rule for psychomotor or temporal lobe epilepsy. There are rare cases involving hypersexuality or perversion but these occur as exceptions in non-psychomotor epilepsy. These findings were confirmed by Earl Walker and Dietrich Blumer (1984, 304, 309).

The absence of sexuality in temporal lobe epilepsy is a basic fact, which bears upon fundamental neuropsychiatric therapy. It means that sexuality and paroxysmality are neurally and biologically distinct. Whereas sexuality seeks preservation of the species and procreation, paroxysmality seeks meaning and value in the face of death. The clarification of these two drive-functions is made clearly and comprehensively by Szondi. This distinction illumines, further, why Arthur Myers was both epileptic and a bachelor, why Frederic Myers' theory of the subliminal self excludes sexuality, and why Dostoevsky's characters lack sustained relationships with women. Prince Myshkin has the gift of foresight and spirituality but knows nothing of women and Kirillov affirms the joy of the aura without child-bearing.

IV. EPILEPSY AND PARANOIA

One of Dostoevsky's original insights dealt with paranoia as a derivative of epilepsy, occurring either after or between seizures. Beginning in 1944, Szondi explored the relationship between epilepsy and paranoia, and he provided detailed documentation of the clinical evidence. In 1895 A. Bucholtz described chronic paranoia on an epileptic base in his *Habilitation* thesis. Seven years later, W. Weygand stated that the epileptic could suffer delusional persecutions and hallucinations. When documenting these early sources, Szondi points out that paranoia strikes after epileptic convulsions have been controlled medically (1963, 278). Similarly, paranoia obtains in stuttering as well as other combinations. As an example, the following paragraph is my translation of one of Szondi's cases (198).

For many years [he] treated a 25-year old, unmarried woman, who suffered genuine epilepsy severely. She lived with her mother, who was a charming but pathologically masochistic, hysterical, and occasionally depressed person. Mother and daughter lived in a sadomasochistic bond. The daughter, who played the sadistic role against the hysterical-masochistic mother in this relationship, attempted to poison her with Luminal. She had to be hospitalized from time to time, because of other paranoid, persecution delusions toward the mother.

Szondi approaches this paranoia-epilepsy link in terms of the theory of ego splitting. For example, inflation might be present in the conscious foreground of the personality, while paroxysmal reactions rumble in the unconscious background. Persons who suffer this kind of splitting display a rapid rotation of these "split-off" phases. So at one time, they become schizoform-inflative, as though possessed, and, at another, they discharge epileptiform seizures in the form of poriomania, which is an aimless, lonely, wandering without any awareness. Dostoevsky portrays this type of splitting in the prodromata and inter-seizure behavior of Prince Myshkin. Szondi contends that rotating ego phases could be exchanged for one another, succeed one another, or work together as opposites (e.g. projective paranoia co-acting with convulsion and violent intent).

The issue discussed by Szondi also raises a historical problem. In 1963 two British psychiatrists presented the same idea, claiming to have achieved a breakthrough. Conceptualized as "the schizophrenic-like psychoses of epilepsy," the study was based upon 69 epileptics, suffering chronic psychoses with grand mal, petit mal, and focal seizures (Slater and Beard 1963). The patients acquired epilepsy in their late teens or early 20s and exhibited auras, twilight states, warm feelings, irritability, aggressiveness, stubbornness, and periodic depression. Despite delusions and hallucinations, the patients retained clear dream content and religious feelings. One of the crucial contributions of this study was the observation that psychoses of epilepsy are cyclical and without mental deterioration. In contrast, genuine schizophrenia runs a course, leading toward mental deterioration. Otherwise, the study did not achieve a breakthrough; for the authors neglected the French and German literature of the asylum doctors. The failure to maintain historical scholarship has been one of the consequences of medical specialization in the age of neurology.

The relationship between epilepsy and paranoia has a fundamental bearing upon this book. As explained primarily by Szondi, paranoia is characterized by the expansion of the ego onto a cosmic level. The paranoid has the unique ability to expand ego boundaries by stripping away bodily limitations (Szondi 1987, 290). This capacity for ego-expansion can be constructive or destructive. On the one hand, one can be healthy and of paranoid disposition and achieve metaphysical understanding or paranormal insight. On the other hand, in an unhealthy state the paranoid can acquire schizophrenia and regress to an elemental level of magical-occult thought, suffering delusions and hallucinations, and sometimes epileptiform symptoms like migraines and stuttering.

V. EPILEPSY, DREAMS, AND DEATH

One of the possible effects of a functional paroxysmal-paranoia is an enhanced psychic sensitivity, including telepathy and clairvoyance. Although this is implied in Frederic Myers' theory of the subliminal self, it is difficult to find the topic discussed in the clinical literature. So I conclude this chapter by presenting a personal situation. In the spring of 1991 I was contacted by a young, white woman who had dreamed of a deceased relative and who wanted an opinion from me on the dream. I agreed to talk with her and, while discussing her dream, she happened to say: "I am epileptic." I then inquired about the nature of her epilepsy.

In early November, 1981, she suffered an automobile accident, in which her head went through the front windshield. About six weeks later, she had a massive grand mal seizure. Thereafter, she continued having grand mal seizures, each one lasting two days. I understood her condition to be a form of post-traumatic epilepsy, in which the accident activates a hereditary predisposition in the form of threshold genes (Niedermeyer 1984, 112). It is also known that carriers of epileptic threshold genes are accident prone (Hedri 1963).

To understand the apparent genetic etiology, I inquired about her family heredity. She told me that her mother's uncle is a temporal lobe epileptic; this relationship would confer a genetic factor of one eighth per cent. Her mother, maternal grandfather, and maternal great-aunt suffered tremors. Her sister had allergies and her son asthma. Her parents had divorced when she was a baby, and she lost contact with her father's family. Nevertheless, the data from the maternal ancestry suggest hereditary factors.

The woman was originally diagnosed in a medical center, given a neurological explanation, and prescribed anticonvulsant medications. I asked her if the neurologist explained the psychological aspects, as known to classical psychiatry, and she said no. Then I explained to her those aspects, which she recognized in herself. The following three paragraphs condense the information she provided me.

She feels pent-up emotion, has a periodic discharge of anger, and yet has acute ethical and religious interests, as well as psychic abilities of clairvoyance and telepathy. Her writing expresses a detailed, round-about style. Interpersonally, she tends toward clinging. After seizures, she feels sluggish, with a sense of heaviness and thickness in the body. She is intolerant of alcohol and, when drinking, becomes dyslectic. She is afraid of eating alone. Finally, she is left-handed and believes herself to be accident prone. These secondary characteristics emerged about two years after the initial grand mal convulsion.

The epileptic attacks come, when sleeping or relaxed. Her grand mal seizures evoke violent convulsions, falling backwards into a dark tunnel, and becoming numb; she hears but cannot respond, yet has a pleasant feeling. When the seizure has ended, she feels tired, sad, and melancholy, having bodily bruises and soreness in the jaw. She then falls into a deep sleep and awakens with the sense of having been dead. Her awakening is a return to reality. Between seizures she sits with a blank stare and exhibits automatisms.

She suffered grand mal seizures for five years, 1981-1986. At the time of my interview, she had not had a seizure for five years. She credited this fact to the anticonvulsant medication but when discussing her medication, I asked if she dreamed. She seemed somewhat surprised by my question but described a specific pattern. Nearly every night she dreams of grinding her teeth, breaking the teeth, spitting them into her hand, and waking up with pain in her jaws. Sometimes, she screams and fears choking, on awakening.

I suggested that the dreams of grinding teeth were focal epileptiform seizures going on despite medication. Contrary to the neurological position, her inner life exhibited the classical symptoms of genuine epilepsy. Further evidence obtains from the fact that prior to the automobile accident in 1981, she had a paranoid tendency. Two years later, when the secondary traits of epilepsy appeared, her paranoid tendency deepened and turned into a paranormal, psychic sensitivity. This development supports Szondi's interpretation of the ego expansiveness of paranoia.

Now as a psychic and epileptic, she perceives auras in people, but they are manifest as heat intensities rather than as colors. She recalled that about 1982 or 1983, she "saw" the "ghost" of her husband's grandfather in the form of a shadow. This presence followed her around the house, but when she said, "go away," it vanished. I asked her about her grandfather's mode of death, and she replied that it was unexpected but could not give details.

Throughout 1987-1988, she beheld the presence of a deceased, elderly female, walking through the house which she and her husband rented. Apparently, the deceased woman was the grandmother of the owner of the house. On three occasions, the lights in the house turned off, while the television was running.

The final evidence of her psychic ability came out during the dream, which prompted her initial contact of me. I suggested that she write about the dream, and I quote her statement below:

[She] was awakened from sleep to find a lady standing next to my bed. This was a very pretty lady with medium length brown hair. She was maybe in her early 30s. She told me that she was very close to J. (my mother in law) and that she needed to reach her and she was having trouble. In a movie type picture in my brain she showed me pictures of my husband's family sometime ago.

The woman in the dream is K., a cousin of the dreamer, who died of cancer in her early 30s and who was a distant acquaintance of the dreamer. The dream came as a surprise.

The scene in the dream shifted to a past time, when a picture appeared of a lady in a hospital type bed with my mother in law standing over the lady and J. was crying. The lady was very sick [and] dark under the eyes, hair very short different style.

This scene reenacts the time when K. was dying.

Then the dream jumps back to the present. K. and the dreamer both leave the latter's house and travel to J.'s house. The dreamer believes that she has left her body and gone to J.'s house with K.. She continues:

> I remember looking down at my feet (bare) and seeing 2 pair of shoes with the soles walked down and 2 pair of white sneakers stepped out of one after another. Then we started through the house and up the stairs. She made it with great ease getting ahead of me. She said that she could reach C. [J.'s husband] but that it was J. that she wanted to talk to.

Halfway up the stairs the dreamer stops and tells K. that she is worried about her children and should return home. K. becomes angry and then reveals her name to the dreamer, who replies that she has never met her. Finally, K. urges the dreamer to tell J. to think of her.

On awakening at 1:00 a.m., the dreamer finds her daughter crying because she had fallen out of bed. When morning came, the woman went to J.'s house and learned that J. had also been awake at 1:00 a.m.. The woman discovered that the shoes in J.'s house belonged to her children and were lying on the floor, exactly as portrayed in the dream. The apparent intent of K.'s appearance in the dream was to contact J., whose children were seriously ill. However, J. was not receptive psychically but the epileptic woman was. Ironically, J. had the following dream a short time later in January, 1991:

> J. is in a room full of people. Some she knows; some she does not know. K. is on the opposite side of the room, looking toward J.. J. did not look in her direction, because she knew K. was dead. J. tried not to look at K. out of fear.

From the perspective of Frederic Myers, the first dream manifests an authentic "phantasm of the dead," whereby the deceased initiates a relation to whomever is sensitive in the family (1903/1954, I, 51). The epilepsy activates the subliminal awareness, which extends across the familial continuum, including the living and the dead.

On September 4, 1991 I presented this case to one of my classes, in order to illustrate the persistence of epileptiform seizures even with anticonvulsants. After class an African student came forward and said that whenever he has the same dream of grinding the teeth and so on, someone in his family dies. Previously, he had the dream four times and, on each occasion, a relative died. I asked if he were epileptic and he said no but his nephew is. His nephew suffers attacks, foaming at the mouth, grinding teeth, and falling—sometimes into a fire. I replied that he is surely a carrier of the genetic predisposition toward epilepsy.

This classroom situation illustrates the fact that bearers of epileptic genes, whether manifest or not, share a basic identity that goes beyond gender, racial, and cultural boundaries. These two persons are gene relatives who relate to each other unconsciously but at a distance as strangers. The fact of gene relatedness also means that genes are dynamic factors in the unconscious.

CHAPTER TWO:
A DYNAMIC ANCESTRY

I. THE FAMILIAL UNCONSCIOUS

Frederic Myers formulated the theory of the subliminal self on the eve of new developments in psychology, neurology, and biology. One of the new movements, in the early twentieth century, was depth psychology, which posited the reality of the unconscious. Sigmund Freud is commonly credited with discovering the unconscious; however, our investigation has revealed that the idea of the unconscious was already implied in Myers' theory of the subliminal self. Furthermore, introspective statements by his brother Arthur demonstrate that he uncovered the existence of the personal unconscious, by reflecting on his petit mal epileptic seizures, which he suffered prior to 1874. As quoted in chapter one, Arthur Myers identified recollection as central to the seizure and that recollection realizes what "has been familiar, but has been for a time forgotten, and now is recovered."

Arthur Myers' statement anticipates exactly Freud's description of the unconscious. In a memorandum to the British Society for Psychical Research, written in 1912, Freud defined the unconscious as follows:

A conception—or any other mental element—which is now *present* to my consciousness may become *absent* the next moment, and may become *present again*, after an interval, unchanged, and, as we say, from memory, not as a result of a fresh perception by our senses.

In the same context Freud goes on to say that an "unconscious concept is one of which we are not aware, but the existence of which we are nevertheless ready to admit on account of other proofs or signs" (Freud 1958, S.E. XII, 260). The unconscious carries material either temporarily forgotten or repressed, which complements gaps in consciousness. The essence of the unconscious consists of instinctual representations that tend to be discharged as wishes (Freud 1957, S.E. XIV, 186). Instinctual drives are signified by the satisfaction of wishes in dreams and neuroses.

Freud conceived of the human organism as a closed system with a finite and unchanging quantity of life energy called libido. He thought of the unconscious as an urge with neither proportionate conflict nor opposites. The urge is a force of essentially sexual material flowing into consciousness and threatening the person, so that it must be expelled from the mind, or repressed. Repression is due to censorship of conflicting feelings that arise particularly from the Oedipus Complex, defined as the son who loves the mother and hates the father.

Freud's model of the unconscious grew out of his work in neurology in 1890. At that time a complete picture of the brain was not available, and Freud failed to realize that thought emerges from electrical activity between individual brain cells or neurons. Thought comprises billions of neurons that fire and create their own energies instantaneously. For example, Freud did not connect epilepsy to neural discharges, as Jackson did, but to conflicts in hysteria traceable to an unresolved Oedipus Complex. He assumed that the nervous system is subject to invasion and intrusion by external sources and that these are defended by reflexes. Freud further assumed that nothing can ever be actually lost in the brain, because it creates nothing new and picks up what is discarded in childhood (1957, S.E. XIV, 195).

Freud's fundamental assumptions have been rejected by neurology on the grounds that the brain is an independent, adaptive system, which generates its own information, and that material can be lost (Hobson 1988, 44-45, 60-64). Early childhood memories before age three are often forgotten, because the brain cuts connections laid down near the time of birth in order to adapt to changing environments. The neurological critique of Freud indirectly confirms the character of the subliminal self, which Frederic Myers described as independent and adaptive. Ironically, Frederic Myers offers compelling evidence against one tenet of neurology and in favor of Freud, namely, every act and idea are registered in the universe (1893/1961, 37). This is rooted in the *deja vu* of epilepsy and, as will be discussed in chapter six, the life review of near death experiences.

To a certain extent, the perspective of Frederic Myers was developed by Carl Jung who began his career in psychiatry as a follower of Freud. However, Jung went beyond Freud by recognizing that although repression occurs, it is neither fundamental nor exclusively sexual. Jung said that libido is like energy in physics and that it pervades the entire physical universe as a vast field and is not confined to the physical contours of the brain. Frederic Myers had stated the same idea, using the analogy of the spectrum of light. Against Freud, Jung contended that psychic energy can split into polar processes and unite them into a whole. The reason is that the life energy behaves in the manner of all natural systems as a self-regulating and balancing process. Since the unconscious is a natural system, it is a self-regulating region which balances itself through flowing syntheses of opposites. The unconscious works by automatic compensation. When consciousness becomes too one-sided or rational, the unconscious compensates by generating irrational forces.

Historically, Jung's insight that the unconscious splits into opposites proved to be crucial in the diagnosis of schizophrenia. The schizophrenic presents a polarity of normal and abnormal parts of the self, split off from each other and acting separately. He learned as a young psychiatrist that the normal part, though hidden in the background, communicates through the abnormal part in the foreground. The person behind the symptoms communicates through symbolic language, and the task of the psychiatrist is to discover the personal narrative. Jung's recognition of unconscious polarity and the role of symbolic language was made in the so-called "Babette Case" (1961, 126-127).

Another discovery by Jung was that of the collective unconscious. Just as the brain has evolved and preserved earlier evolutionary eras in its structure, so has the psyche. The psyche or mind comprises a universal awareness that is partly conscious but mainly unconscious and that is an energy field connected to each person through the brain stem. While consciousness serves as the seat of sense perception and the agent of social interaction, the unconscious formulates knowledge. Sensory knowledge consists of mental imagery, because data must be processed through the brain-mind system. As sensory data are processed, they are simultaneously interpreted as symbols. Altogether, the psyche encompasses sensory processing in the brain and symbol formation in the mind.

Jung illustrates these functions with a common example. He notes that to the open vision of the eye the sun appears to rise every morning, ascend to a mid-day peak, and then descend to darkness at sunset. This obvious and daily sighting of the sun, repeated since primeval times, also registers in the mind, where it is interpreted in a symbolic form. By analogy, the psyche symbolizes the rising and the setting of the sun as the cycle of human existence. So in the morning or childhood, life arises and ascends to the peak of consciousness and then, at mid-day or noon, descends through aging and suffering to death or the unconscious. Thus, what the eye sees becomes through the mind the universal model of living and dying.

However, Jung extended the symbol of the sun's arc into a model of self-development and grounded it in the hero myth. The person like the hero takes consciousness away from the mother and develops in a linear manner into adulthood and self-consciousness. At the midpoint of life, the person begins to feel the pull of death and so, in the second half, descends to death or returns to the unconscious. In the second half of life one does not grow in linear phases but by dramatic breakthroughs that deepen consciousness and prepare for death. Clearly, the hero myth goes beyond the basic cross-over pattern of the sun, and Jung's interpretation will be opposed by an appeal to archeology in chapter three and to Ancient Near Eastern mythology in chapter seven.

According to Jung, the collective unconscious contains instinctual drives and archetypes. Instinctual drives are unconscious, inherited, and uniform motivations of behavior. They are automatic, necessary, but not creative. Jung lists the drives in terms of their biological primacy. (1) Hunger is the first one, followed by (2) sexuality. When these two are satisfied, then (3) a drive to activity emerges, followed by (4) a reflective and (5) a creative drive which is capable of suppressing the others (1960, 116-118). Jung's scheme is questionable logically and biologically. Citing a creative drive is contradicted by the prior definition that a drive is not creative. Further, these drives are stated without reference to animal studies, which would demonstrate a genetic homology between animal and human functions. Jung also fails to provide an assessment of the tensions of the drives, their variabilities and modes of satisfaction. Finally, Jung omits the startle network of the brain, the paroxysmal pattern, according to which every animal and every human being are susceptible to a seizure in response to irritation or shock (Niedermeyer 1984, 112). The apparent reason for his neglect of epilepsy is that he makes schizophrenia the paradigmatic disease.

The archetypes are innate, preformed dispositions which strive for manifestation in conscious life. Archetypes do not appear directly but indirectly as symbols, since they remain unconscious. Archetypes are reflexive forms that evolve from the unconscious, just as seeds grow into trees. Although archetypes tend toward the goal of manifestation, they erupt in the manner of volcanic upheavals. Similarly, instinctual drives also erupt from the unconscious. Both drives and archetypes discharge the universal psychic energy through their respective incursions.

Jung imagined the collective unconscious to be like a vast ocean, on the surface of which mountain summits are visible as a result of volcanic explosions. Similarly, James and Myers compared the subliminal self to the ocean. Jung also used a geographical model, when he portrayed, in a 1925 lecture published posthumously, the following unconscious layers in the evolutionary psyche: families, clans, nations, large groups (e.g. Europeans), primate ancestors, animal ancestors, and the hidden fire as background radiation of all cosmic origins (1925/1989, 134). The hidden fire would be interpreted in contemporary physics as the residual radiation, emanating from the explosive origin of the universe called the "Big Bang."

These layers are listed without a framework of an evolving hierarchy in the universe. Jung does not clearly distinguish between ancestral and collective content, as he admits in his autobiography (1961, 233, 237). In his view, archetypes are models deployed by the ancestors and transmitted to descendants. In a lecture delivered on April 20, 1925, Jung asserts that one may become possessed by an ancestor. Conceding that this idea is hypothetical, lacking scientific evidence, Jung goes on to say "that these ideas of ancestor possession would be that these autonomous complexes exist in the mind as Mendelian units, which are passed on from generation to generation intact, and are unaffected by the life of the individual" (1925/1989, 37). He explains that analysis tries to discover the ancestral traits and assimilate them with consciousness. Jung's appeal to genetics or "Mendelian units" is promising, but the idea confuses genes with psychological concepts of complex and possession. In retrospect, had Jung been able to conceptualize a distinct genetics of the unconscious, he would have made a fundamental conceptual advance beyond Myers.

Meanwhile in Budapest, Szondi began his pioneering investigations of the family and made seminal contributions to psychiatric genetics, as noted in chapter one. His early research was governed by the assumption that a psychic trait equals one or more genes. Through extensive pedigree studies Szondi found that genetically-induced traits are manifest, particularly in basic decision-making. By laying out a family tree, it would be possible to trace unconscious genetic influences in mate and vocational selection, as well as other existential choices. The sources of decisions could be derived neither from repressed wishes nor from collective archetypal representations. After examining several hundred genealogies, he published an English language essay in 1937, demonstrating genetic influences in marriage choice. The following is one example:

> *Case 21.* A woman, cook on a ship, makes the acquaintance of a reckless gambler on the ship, and falls in love with him. Later they get married. They have a daughter who is epileptic. The husband is killed in the gambling club. After the death of her husband she enters a concubinage with a labuorer [sic] in brickworks, from whom she has three children. One of these, a girl, is also epileptic (Szondi 1937, 46).

The woman has given birth to two epileptic children by two different men. Viewed relationally, all three are gene relatives. Since the men are not identified as manifest epileptics, then they must be carriers of genes for the disease. Thus, the case indicates that epilepsy is recessive. Consequently, to acquire the disease one must inherit one gene for epilepsy from each parent. Should one inherit one epileptic gene that is paired with a normal gene, then receiving a single-dosage gene makes one a carrier, who does not become epileptic. Szondi contends that the single-dosage genes, carried by the woman and her two partners, are the source of their mutual attraction. As a consequence of their respective matings, two epileptic children are born.

The case continues, and I quote the remainder:

> The daughter from the first (and legitimate) marriage had once a bad quarrel with her husband, seized an axe in her anger and

threatened him with it; but afterwards she fainted and had typical epileptic fits. These fits return since regularly. This daughter bore eleven children, among them three epileptic and one eclamptic. The second daughter from the concubinage got married too and had a child who died in eclamptic cramps.

The first daughter acquired her epilepsy after a fit of anger, which confirms Szondi's theory that the seizure is a defense against the Cain homicidal intent (1969, 53-54). Pent-up emotion causes the recessive epileptic genes to penetrate the phenotype. This epileptic gave birth to three epileptic children and one eclamptic child. This presupposes her mating with a bearer of one or two epileptic genes. In classical psychiatry eclampsia is regarded as a paroxysmal equivalent of epilepsy. So of the 11 children four are born with paroxysmal-epileptiform disturbances. This ratio of four out of 11 conforms to the percentages of transmission in classical Mendelian genetics, namely: 25% chance of being effected by the disease; 50% chance of acquiring the gene in single-dosage and becoming a carrier; and 25% of being totally uneffected. Finally, the case illustrates the distinction between blood relatives and gene relatives. Marriage among blood relatives is prohibited by the incest taboo, but in actual practice mate selection occurs by means of mutual attraction among gene relatives (Szondi 1937, 71).

In a subsequent essay, recently reprinted, Szondi argues that heredity influences choice behavior in terms of opposites (1955/1992, 22-25). The reason is that genetic information is transmitted on genes and chromosomes from mother and father. Such dual heredities make polarity inherent in genetic transmission. In cases of psychopathology the genetic predisposition is manifest both as a trait and as a defense against it. Manifestation of the trait takes place as the striving of a need, which simultaneously triggers a defense as a means of satisfaction. In the case of the epileptic daughter, cited above, she feels anger and picks up an axe ready to kill. Since she is threatened by the fit, she defends against it by fainting and undergoing epileptic convulsions. Her epileptic attack is a defense against the need to kill in the form of the "death-feigning reflex" (*Totstellreflex*).

The case of epilepsy helps to reveal, further, the nature of the familial unconscious. Genuine epileptic convulsions appear only from time to time. Meanwhile, as the asylum doctors knew, the epileptic behaves differently as implied in the notion of masked epilepsy. Between seizures one feels religious, acts morally, or becomes psychically sensitive. Szondi contends that behavior between attacks is also governed by epileptic genes which are hidden in the genotype. The same may be said of schizophrenia or manic-depression. Because of the alternating phases of these genetically-based psychopathologies, Szondi developed the concept of psychic rotation, using the image of a revolving stage. As a stage, the personality is driven to turn around; suddenly the background rotates into the foreground and vice versa. Psychic rotation parallels the established genetic fact of dominance variability, which means that most variations occur with dominant genes (Milunsky 1989, 97).

Since everyone becomes shocked or angry but is not epileptic, this raises even further the question of variability. Along with the polarity of heredity, Szondi conceives of a latent proportionality in the familial unconscious. The dual paternal and maternal heredities vary with respect to intensity. Every person bears instinctual drives, and heredity determines the relative range of intensity of each of the drives. Szondi differentiates between three drive centers in the animal brain: sexual, paroxysmal, and contact, which is the drive to make and maintain relationships, as exemplified in attachment behavior. The ego is added in the system, but it derives exclusively from the human levels of the brain. No rigorous determinism is entailed, because genes interact with the environment through the drives, and these are modulated by the ego. The interaction involves a range of drive-needs, which may be normal or abnormal.

The fact of genetic variability leads to an even further aspect of the familial unconscious, namely, heterosis or high Darwinian vitality. Heterosis means that, in the case of recessives, carriers of the genes in single-dosage are heterozygous and, consequently, healthier and stronger than those who receive a double-dosage of the gene. The latter are homozygotic recessive, and they acquire the trait. The fact of heterosis was originally established in clinical observations that male heterozygotes have more mating speed in courtship compared to male homozygotes. Theodosius Dobzhansky explains that sexually and out breeding species have high rates of heterozygosis, including humans (1970, 178-198). The reason, he suggests, is that heterosis is one way of balancing adaptations of organisms and environments and of guaranteeing genetic variability. The notion of heterosis depends on the existence of recessive genes, whose traits are believed to be negative or ambiguous. The recessives arise by mutation and remain as genetic loads to populations until they pass out by natural selection. However, negative recessives leave gene pools no more rapidly than so-called positive genes. There is no ideal typology of normal genes, from which recessive mutants deviate. Rather, recessives balance genetic loads by yielding more vital offspring, who in turn facilitate adaptation. Thus, heterozygotes have a higher reproductive input into populations.

Early investigators established that carriers of the gene for sickle cell anemia in single-dosage are healthy and resistant to malaria (Milunsky 1989, 117). Carriers of a cystic fibrosis recessive gene seem to be immune to influenza and possibly cholera (Harris and Super 1987, 73). Cystic fibrosis does not follow the classical Mendelian percentages, but it varies in different ways: 66% for full sibling; 50% for half sibling; and 50% for sister or brother with cystic offspring. The cystic gene is located on the long arm of chromosome #11.

Heterotic balancing is discussed in several places in Szondi's writings. In an early essay he assesses the original experimental evidence of heterosis and argues for a revision of the notion of genetic load. Instead of viewing the genetic load as purely negative, he recommends the conception of a familial load (*familiären Belastung*), which means that descendants of genetically-ill ancestors receive vitality that defends against the negative traits in constructive social roles (Szondi 1949, 11). The familial load of genetically-tainted families motivates the selection of socially positive vocations.

Throughout his extensive writings, Szondi employs the German adjective *familiäre* to mean "familial." His German usage presupposes the same in Latin, where *familiaris* means "family" or "household." Family members are familiars in classical usage. The familial load is essentially the same as the familial unconscious, and it covers two kinds of relationships. One is that of blood relatedness, traceable through paternal and maternal ancestry, and the other is that of gene relationships, whereby choices of mates, friends, and vocations are influenced by genetic dispositions. Persons chosen by genetic tendencies are also familiars. The familial unconscious is an overlapping band of generations, a "vertical" stream of blood relatives and a "horizontal" stream of gene relatives (Bürgi-Meyer 1987, 10).

A well known example of gene-relatedness and vocational selection is that those with a disposition toward schizophrenia choose psychiatry as a vocational outlet. Choosing this helping profession balances the deleterious gene for schizophrenia in the familial load. The current situation in American psychiatry illustrates this issue. E. Fuller Torrey chose psychiatry as his profession because, when he was 19 years old, his 17 year old sister became schizophrenic with a paranoid psychosis. She began to hear hallucinatory voices, and consequently, he believes that hearing voices is the central symptom of schizophrenia in 75% of patients (Dajer 1992, 43). Torrey is the leading exponent of the viral theory of schizophrenia, and he acknowledges that the aural hallucination indicates damage in the left temporal lobe of the brain.

In summary, the familial unconscious, as described by Szondi comprises a (1) polar, (2) genetically proportionate, and (3) heterotic balancing structure. The notion of familial or familiarity extends an original insight of Arthur Myers, who uncovered, through recollections, forgotten material that was familiar (Jackson 1931, 401). Freud did not advance decisively beyond the Myers' brothers mutual articulation of the unconscious, since he mainly detected the dynamic force of repression. Carl Jung actually continued along the lines of Frederic Myers' vision but innovated with his discovery of polarity. Only Szondi advanced beyond Myers with his discovery of the genetics of the unconscious.

However, in light of Szondi's genetics studies, we may pose a question to Carl Jung. Why does the unconscious split into opposites? The answer is that one receives two heredities from two parents, in which the "ladder" structure of the DNA molecule possesses a polar form and the genes are arranged contiguously on the two "sides of the ladder." The coded information yields dual forms in the drives of the organism.

If one were to ask how the familial unconscious could be known, the answer would come from therapy. One of Szondi's dramatic cases deals with a male patient, whose genealogy carries several epileptic and paranoid relatives. For example, his mother suffers migraines, and her father had had epilepsy since age 15. A sister of the maternal grandfather is schizophrenic. The father has fits of rage and poriomania. Two maternal cousins are paranoid psychotic. The patient, however, is neither epileptic nor paranoid, as such. Psychological testing reveals manifest sexual disturbance and interpersonal instability. These conditions occupy the foreground, and the epileptic and paranoid traits linger in the background by virtue of his heredity.

In the course of therapy the patient displays symptoms of an epileptic aura. He feels sick, seems to be sinking into a nothingness, gets anxiety over the impending attack. He moans, gasps for air, and exhibits the symptoms of asthma. He wants to jump off the couch, attack his therapist violently, and run out of the room in an epileptic fugue. With the seizure he has hysterical struggles of laughing and weeping; hallucinations and illusions; paranoid guilt; persecution fantasies and delusions (Szondi 1955/1992, 21). Metaphorically, his epileptic and paranoid relatives have returned in a moment of shock suffering.

This therapeutic episode not only attests to the familial unconscious but also to the fact that pathological symptoms derive from the genotype rather than the archetypes. The sudden turn-around, springing the relatives' traits into view, so to speak, gives evidence that the mental threshold pertains to genes as well as to consciousness. As Szondi has shown convincingly, the threshold is indeed variable and it can be raised or lowered in accordance with the degree of genetic penetration. Whether one possesses a predisposition or even manifests the trait in the phenotype makes little difference genetically. The ancestors are always standing backstage, ready to rush onto the stage of the mind. They are strange but familiar characters.

II. THREE LANGUAGES OF DISEASE

Szondi's discovery of the familial unconscious was not intended to displace the significant contributions of Freud and Jung but to integrate them. Altogether the unconscious or subliminal self comprises distinct and co-active personal, collective, and familial regions. Szondi has described the unconscious as a poly-functional system (1955/1992, 8), in which each domain speaks its own "language:" symptom (personal), symbol (collective), and decision (familial).

As an illustration of these three languages, terminal cancer is considered. In contemporary clinical experience cancer is the paradigm of fatal illness, because it flourishes in epidemic proportions, particularly in affluent societies. Normally, cancer emerges from a long, slow, and hidden incubation process and, even after its onset, creates unique images that amplify the character of the symptoms. Imagery helps the patient cope with the disease and filter treatment decisions. Images take shape as metaphors, through which the patient expresses self-understanding and anxiety. Cancer metaphors retain binding force, because they bring some degree of control to a disease with an ineradicable mystery (Sontag 1978, 5-6). The more mysterious a disease, the more is imagery needed for coping with the shame, fear, and dread. Cancer is as mysterious as epilepsy, and the metaphors of epilepsy express eruptive, elemental forces, such as fire, ocean waves, and earthquakes. Cancer metaphors express the body under attack, besieged, aggressive cell growth, tormented by degeneration of the flesh, horrible pain, dread of soiling, and dirt.

Psychoanalysis has pioneered in the study of this disease, mainly because Freud died of cancer in 1939. Since he described the unconscious with intrusive and invasive notions, which are cancer metaphors, was his theory shaped by the incubation of his own illness? Psychoanalysis examines how the disease intrudes from within, invading the unconscious layers of the organism, and how it activates corresponding images. It also exposes the psychodynamic process behind the cancer metaphors.

Although there are many kinds of cancer, at issue psychoanalytically is whether the disease takes a tumor or a nontumor form. Gotthard Booth developed a profile that has become useful in approaching the tumor patient (1979, 99-100): (1) He or she suffers the imprinting of a trauma in the first few years of life, creating a lack of basic trust. (2) Out of the trauma comes a life-long need for control. (3) The disease eventually sets in, when one loses control over a particular "object," usually after a serious loss. (4) The disease locates in the organ that dominates the genetic make-up of the person and the lost "object." This point implies that the strongest, central, or controlling organ in one's life suffers the illness. (5) The tumor symbolizes the lost "object," so that, through the disease one holds onto it unconsciously. (6) The course of the disease depends upon whether one surrenders the "object" and works through the loss, or whether one resists and retains the "object" as an unconscious source of pleasure. Working through promotes healing, resistance encourages the disease.

Booth emphasizes that disease is not evil but is a revelation of one's limits and one-sidedness. Underlying the psychoanalytic profile are the dynamics of depression, specifically futile clinging to a lost "object." Sometimes, the tumor represents the negative aspect of a person in one's life, such as, for example, the mother of a breast cancer patient who also died of breast cancer (Dreifuss-Kattan 1990, 162-163). A personified tumor introduces a splitting within the self, so that the patient may either project or introject the "object." The tumor is a thing that expands, as a non-self entity, amorally and asocially. Projection is frequently accompanied by denial, particularly in the early phases of the disease. Denial conserves the status quo, protects the self from disintegration, and offers a sense of control. Denial may be expressed through projection as an irrational falsification of the condition or as a cheery optimism. When these prove to be unsuccessful, the tumor patient may introject the tumor as a bad thing, which cannot be eliminated. This would lower self-worth and facilitate depression. In death the bad thing triumphs inside.

When cancer takes a nontumor form, as in leukemia, the patient cannot dwell on a thing, a split-off nonself within. Unable to project or introject an "object," the patient is flooded with high fever, physical weakness, and fear, which threaten psychic disintegration. In order to cope, the patient may view the care-giver as healthy and whole, with whose self-image he or she wishes to identify; yet this wish has to be denied (ibid., 191). By fusing with the healthy care-giver, the patient incorporates a new identity and doubles the self. Through doubling one narcissistically inflates oneself into a new and healthy being. While this inflation might temporarily defend against the dread of the disease, eventually it breaks down, and the patient sees his or her own sickness mirrored in the concerns of the care-giver. When the fusion leads to realistic mirroring, the fear of death surfaces. The patient then becomes vulnerable to the dual images of sickness and health, life and death, being and nonbeing. One becomes victim to a primal agony and fears falling into a state of disintegration. Whereas the fear of falling echoes the dread of epilepsy, the dynamics of fusing, doubling, and mirroring may occur with AIDS patients as well.

Further, the Jungian view of cancer is well represented in a paper by Russell Lockhart (1977). He states correctly that our word symptom derives from two Greek roots: *syn*, which means "together," and *pitein*, which means "to fall." He interprets symptom to mean two or more things that fall together, as though by chance. Thus, when cancer strikes, one feels victimized by random forces for which one is not responsible (13). Feeling victimized and out of control induces a splitting within the self. Lockhart's interpretation reflects Jung's insight that cancer befalls the extrovert who, while investing energy in external structures, becomes stuck internally and ceases to grow. This dilemma of the extrovert is partially established collectively and psychically by industrial society, whose alienation from nature serves as a breeding ground for cancer. In contrast, cancer is virtually absent in undeveloped, tribal society, which is more closely related to nature.

In the collective unconscious cancer stimulates the imagination. Lockhart states the well-known etymology of symbol. The Greek prefix *syn* combines with the infinitive *ballein*, which means "to throw." Hence, symbol implies two things thrown together intentionally to produce the meaning. He illustrates the etymology with the case of a dying woman who, unexpectedly and spontaneously, painted a crocodile holding a clock. In the painting she "threw together" a reptile and a machine, announcing from her unconscious, animal nature: "Your time has come" to die.

Generally, cancer images represent natural forces of predatory aggression. The body is being torn in two, consumed, and assaulted. Cancer belongs to that part of the self that is denied, undernourished, cut down, and unable to grow. Cancer images frequently convey motifs involving earth and plants, such as cutting down trees or crossing a field as a stranger. These may accompany feelings of guilt and retribution, promises to change and make sacrifices, while doing nothing at all.

Finally, cancer betrays hereditary patterns. When viewed from the perspective of the familial unconscious, Szondi's extensive pedigree studies have confirmed that certain families bear specific inclinations toward terminal illness. This fact pertains both to cancer as a hereditary disease and to its bodily location. The following quotation is my translation of one example:

> In one case the mother died of uterine and breast cancer, the father of a stroke. Of the twelve surviving children two sons remain free of cancer. Three of the daughters died of uterine cancer, one of ovarian, and two of breast cancer. Thus, five daughters followed their mother with respect to the organ attacked by the disease, so that one may speak of a kind of "organ choice." Of the grandchildren one died again of breast cancer, another of uterine, and the third (a man) of bowel cancer (Szondi 1987, 359).

Such familial patterns provide a genetic foundation to the psychoanalytically observed fact of organ choice in cancer patients. They cohere with the existence of proto-oncogenes, which numbering about forty, are activated by specific enzymes; thereby becoming oncogenes which then make cells cancerous. Cancer cells reproduce themselves indefinitely through abnormal growth. Abnormal cell growth corresponds to the image of cancer in ancient Greek medicine, namely, the crab that creeps in unpredictable, sideways motions at night. Like the crab cancer is an aggressive, unassailable force that inflicts pain and threatens death.

III. CONCEPT OF GENOTROPISM

The familial unconscious is governed by polarity, latent proportionality, and heterotic balancing selection, but the operating mechanism is called genotropism. Genotropism is defined as a reciprocal attraction between carriers of related or identical genes (Szondi 1987, 41). The concept of genotropism grew out of Szondi's early family studies (1937) and was formally presented in a lecture in Geneva, Switzerland (1939, 45). He intended the notion of genotropism to be the psychological version of classical Mendelian genetics. Since classical genetics dealt with dominant and recessive modes of transmission, these factors shaped the original formulation of the concept. Consequently, in many case studies Szondi demonstrated that carriers of latent recessive genes tend to become attracted to one another. Carrying the gene of a specific trait was the motivation for choice behavior and heterosis.

Since the 1930s, many advances have been made in biology; and so it is necessary to consider genotropism, not only in terms of recessives but also in light of dominants, sex-linked, chromosomal aberrations, and so forth. While investigations continue, the basic issue is whether genes for specific traits surpass a threshold, penetrate the phenotype, and influence choice behavior. The fact of genetic influence on decision-making can be established by detecting relationships in genealogies. Certain genes co-exist with certain patterns of choice; for example, epilepsy, migraines, and stuttering in families of religious professions.

The concept of genotropism remains controversial, especially in European psychiatry where it is better known. One of the common objections to the concept is that genes are static and not dynamic. Szondi has argued, in reply, that genes are active in psychopathology (1955/1992, 23). Whoever has encountered the force of epileptic seizures, schizophrenic neologisms, and manic-depressive psychoses, has experienced the dynamics of genes.

The active nature of genes has been confirmed by the concept of genesmanship, according to which genes facilitate their own survival by replicating multiple copies of themselves and by creating cooperation among their carriers (Dawkins 1976, 97). Genes undergo natural selection, and their goal is to survive in subsequent generations. Evolving organisms have the ability to detect similar genes in others and to select them for mating and reproduction. Mating with people of related or identical genetic traits increases the number of shared genes in the offspring by 50%. Experimental studies indicate that couples married for four years have more genes in common than do those who divorce earlier (Bereczkei 1992, 37-39). These factors validate genetropism. Normally, attraction takes place through the face, as carriers reflect their genetic traits by expression, cues, or feelings. In the case of blindness, attraction also operates, and this indicates that the medium of the attraction is truly unconscious.

Genotropism operates in five areas of human experience (Szondi 1987,57): (1) Genotropism conditions choices of love and marriage partners, who are attracted to and remain bonded with each other. (2) Genotropism informs selection of friends and ideas, thus shaping common interest groups. (3) It works in vocational choices. (4) Genes that influence the foregoing healthy choices mutate to condition illness and (5) death, as already indicated.

To illustrate some forms of genotropism even further, the eminent persons discussed in chapter one may be reconsidered. Arthur Myers was epileptic, and his brother Frederic a pioneer in the psychology of death and psychic activities. It is highly probable that Frederic was a carrier of the genetic predisposition to epilepsy. He conceptualized the subliminal self or unconscious as that which erupts like a seizure in a state of lowered conscious threshold. The genealogy reveals religious professions, which correlate with inherited epilepsy. The father of Arthur and Frederic was an Anglican clergyman, and the paternal ancestry was dominated by clergy. Further, the brothers' friendship choice showed genotropic activity in the sense that Henry Sidgwick, co-founder with Frederic of the Society for Psychical Research, was a stutterer (Murphy and Ballou 1973, 199). Stuttering is a genetic equivalent of epilepsy.

Frederic Myers had a love affair with a maternal cousin named Annie, who was married to a manic-depressive and who had two sisters, one of whom died in a psychosis. The maternal branch of Frederic

Myers' family had many businessmen. In his autobiographical essay (1893/1961) Frederic writes many poems to Annie but disguises her name as Phyllis (Taylor and Marsh 1980, 763). Annie committed suicide by drowning in 1876, and her death compelled Frederic to believe in immortality as a means of restitution. Drowning is a preferred suicide choice of persons with paroxysmal-epileptiform heredity (Szondi 1987, 360). A love affair among first cousins presupposes genotropic attraction, and, in the case of Annie and Frederic, the common genetic factor would probably be the genetic predisposition to epilepsy.

Later in his life Myers claimed that, after he died, he would send messages to the living through a medium. His choice was Lenore Piper, the well-known Boston medium, whose career began with epileptic seizures. There is no proof of post-mortem communication from Myers through Piper, but the fact that he chose her as his ideal is genotropic.

Dostoevsky, it will be recalled, died of tuberculosis in 1881. Likewise, his mother Mariya died of tuberculosis in 1837, as did his first wife, also named Mariya, in 1864. The latter had been married to a teacher, an alcoholic, who died of tuberculosis as well. These genotropic patterns are balanced by the fact that Dostoevsky married his second wife Anna in 1867, and she bore him four children, one of whom, Aleksey, died of an epileptic seizure at age three in 1878. Aleksey's convulsion lasted three hours and ten minutes, and it gave proof to his father of the familial inheritance of epilepsy. Assuming the inheritance to be recessive, then Anna has to be an epileptic carrier.

Therese Wagner-Simon and Irina Haefely-Grauen have sorted out the genetic patterns in a comprehensive study of Dostoevsky's genealogy (1985, 28-29; 1986, 13). Anna inherited a disposition to epilepsy from her mother's family. She displayed distinctive characteristics of the epileptoid personality, such as attention to details, emotional outbursts followed by phases of unclear thinking, and inclination toward clairvoyance. She had precognitive dreams and premonitions, through which she predicted future events. Her gift of foresight derives from epileptoid heredity and is probably the basis for genetic attraction to her husband.

All of the children of Anna and Fyodor suffered scrofula, which is a form of tuberculosis characterized by tumors in the neck that generate pus. This fact suggests a hereditary constitutional type which makes one susceptible to tuberculosis.

IV. PAROXYSMAL DEATH SYMBOLISM

The theory of genotropism logically entails a potentially self refuting dilemma. If genes be active in psychopathology, how may they survive, if they were not reproduced? Ordinarily, mental disorders tend to decrease survival and reproductive success. People with poor mental health either remain unmarried, or, when they marry and bear children, they transmit defective genes to their offspring who risk contracting the illness (Bereczkei 1992, 43).

This issue pertains particularly to epilepsy, which in its genuine psychomotor form discourages sexual interest, arousal, and activity. Obviously, this condition inhibits the possibility of genes for epilepsy surviving. Historically, one resolution of the problem was to sterilize epileptics. Szondi confronted this problem many years ago, when first presenting the concept of genotropism. He appealed to heterosis as a fact and contended that genotropism has two positive features: (1) sublimation in the character and (2) socialization in a vocation (Szondi 1939, 60). With this observation he opposed sterilization and suggested that vocational therapy be used to find socially constructive outlets for those who bear genetic pathological predispositions.

Several years later the same dilemma was faced by William Lennox, who rejected sterilization and even encouraged epileptics to marry (1951, 529). He suggested that epileptics transmit other positive traits but did not specify what they might be. The idea of heterosis means that deleterious genes survive in populations, when they transmit positive traits that outweigh the negative. Heterosis involves a balancing of tendencies among the same genes. With respect to the concept of genesmanship, it is not that similar genes recognize one another but that they achieve an adaptive balance. Just as carriers of genes for schizophrenia produce psychiatrists as socially positive persons, so in the same way do genes for epilepsy create constructive outlets. However, the question arises; what is the genetic advantage of epilepsy?

My contention is that threshold epilepsy defends against the threat of death through sublimation of paroxysmal energy. Essentially, sublimation means that the energy of an instinctual drive is transferred to a higher level to gain greater value. Although the goal be changed, the energy remains the same. The notion of sublimation was originally proposed by Freud, who restricted it to the sexual drive. He argued, for example, that religious and cultural symbolism is sublimated sexuality.

Szondi agreed with Freud's definition of sublimation but applied it to other instinctually driven areas, such as religion and ethics (1977, 150). Szondi grounded sublimation in the biological polarity of heredity or heterosis. On the basis of this biological polarity I argue that the psychologies of death, including mythological and theological forms, are also sublimations of the aggressive energy released in the epileptic seizure.

My argument draws upon the introspective understanding of epilepsy in the classical age of the asylum doctors before the advent of neurology. One source is an anonymous paper written by an epileptic in 1825 and used as a reference in the older psychiatric literature. He describes the sun constantly moving before his eyes and then disappearing; after which a square of light, about four or five feet wide, takes shape around him. Male figures arise from the darkness at the right edge of the light and pass before him into the darkness of the left.

> As I gazed after them, I had a feeling they were my enemies, who had first lain in wait in the darkness and then put a chain around my breast and heart. It seemed to me that they wanted to tear me to pieces with the chain, and I defended myself with all the strength of my body, clenching my teeth, and clasping my hands together (Temkin and Temkin 1968, 567).

Others observed during his epileptic seizure that he had clenched teeth, foam at the mouth, and he uttered a loud cry. Afterward, he felt anxiety, had a headache, and saw spots moving in front of his eyes. This statement reveals the seizure to be a defense against a life-threatening assault, a force of death, as it were, amid proto-symbolic patterns of light and darkness.

A second source comes from the German physiologist Johannes Purkyne, who suffered childhood epilepsy and considered its essence to be dizzy spells or vertigo. On the inside, the vertigo takes symbolic forms and, on the outside, involuntary, violent convulsions, and loss of consciousness. He conceived of epilepsy as involving a relationship between an inner affective disturbance and outer muscular action. Purkyne published introspective, physiological descriptions of epilepsy, and these have been collected by Paul Vogel (1935). I translate below a decisive description of vertigo as expressed in dream symbolization:

where we image ourselves rotating passively and in a whirlpool with dreadful feeling. I suffered eclampsia as a child, from 7-10 years, and clearly remember having a dream symbol. It came to me as an immense, swirling sea of fire, in which I would be turning ever more quickly, and struggle with all my powers, until I lost consciousness. To bystanders these movements appeared externally to be clonic convulsions, even though they would only be a movement of a vertigo dream (Vogel 1935, 229).

Vogel notes that about 1925 research into epilepsy turned away from Purkyne's relational approach to the mechanistic method of Jacksonian neurology.

A third source comes from the biography of Vincent Van Gogh, who was diagnosed as epileptic by doctors at St. Rémy asylum. His seizures lasted for several hours or even weeks, during which he exhibited violent, restless agitation and ecstatic religious visions. The German psychiatrist Walter Riese confirmed the diagnosis of epilepsy and explained how the disease influenced the painter's artistic temperament. Van Gogh struggled "for the essential, the absolute, the simple, the unambiguous in human nature and existence" and, at the same time, had a "dire need of his fellow men and of their love" (Riese 1958, 200). This dialectic of hyperreligiousness and adhesiveness led Van Gogh "to deprive visual objects of all that is merely incidental in order to 'prove' the law which is revealed by the *general* nature of line and colour." As any observer could attest, the inner law of reality, as disclosed by Van Gogh's paintings, is a dynamic vortex, whether in a starry night, wheat fields, or sunflowers. His swirling visual forms are like the auras seen by psychics.

These combined sources cohere with the eruptive symbolizations as described by Frederic Myers: "the scarlet fire of the epileptic," "uprush of the hidden fire," and "earthquake wave of an unfathomed sea." Similarly, Nicolas Berdyaev identifies Dostoevsky's element as fire, his style one of movement, and his characters as victims of underground volcanoes (1957, 20).

Szondi maintained the classical tradition of relational epilepsy but expanded it to include genotropic choice behavior. The genetically-conditioned affective disorders influence corresponding forms of vocational selection:

I. Vocations dominated by sense organs: sense of equilibrium, smell.

II. Vocational motifs, the primal elements: earth, fire, water, air, psyche.

III. Vocational position: height-depth, ascent-descent, whirling motions, undulating, wave-like rhythms (Szondi 1987, 268).

Some examples of these paroxysmal-epileptiform choices are jobs involving vehicles and transportation, such as truck drivers and railroaders. With reference to the elements, we find coal miners (earth), fire fighters (fire), sailors (water), and pilots (air). Under the motif of psyche are the religious and helping professions, such as medicine, law, clinical psychology, and social work, as well as psychic research as distinguished from spiritualism and the occult.

To illustrate even further two examples of selectional patterns and genealogies are translated as follows:

Case 42. Hystero-epileptic, female patient (Szondi 1987, 271-272).

A. Paroxysmal illnesses in the family.

1. A maternal uncle and the first wife of the maternal grandfather were *epileptics*. 2. The mother suffered migraines.

B. Paroxysmal vocations in the family.

1. A brother, who died in an airplane crash, was a *flight-officer*. A brother-in-law was also a *flight-officer*.

Case 44. A female patient travels as a petty thief and *vagabond*, which required her to be institutionalized in a reformatory. (272-273).

A. Paroxysmal illnesses in the family.

1. The mother suffered *migraines*. 2. The brother of the mother was a poriomanic *vagabond*. 3. On account of *arson* the mother's brother, a *butcher's helper* was imprisoned. He later became delusional, possibly a psychotic epileptic. 4. In a violent moment of *passion* the father committed a murder. Because the village notary had insulted him for his *religious* feelings, he shot him.

B. Paroxysmal vocations in the family.

1. A maternal cousin of the patient was a *waiter on an ocean steamer*. 2. A brother as well as his friends were *fire fighters*. Further, a half-brother of the mother later became a *fire chief*.

In Case 44 lighting fires and putting out fires are expressions of the biological polarity of paroxysmal-epileptiform genes. The same dialectic informs murder and the slaughtering of animals for food by the butchers.

The combined case material indicates that the biological polarity has achieved evolutionary stability. Choosing jobs in terms of the primal elements is a constructive socialization of the genetic root. On the basis of the same root all humans symbolize the shock of death through motifs of height and depth, ascent and descent, vortex and undulating process, as well as the primal elements of air, earth, water, fire, and psyche.

CHAPTER THREE:
SYMBOL OF THE TRANSPERSONAL
SELF

I. THE PONTIFICAL EGO

Although humankind inherits a dynamic ancestry, life is not strictly determined. Humans are essentially free beings, who can accept or reject familial patterns. Certainly in cases of hereditary mental disorders persons are driven to act out compulsively the morbid traits of their ancestors. Ironically, psychopathology involves behavior whose intent is to grasp freedom from unconscious conflicts in any way possible. This normally includes substitutionary modes of behavior that may appear to be liberating but in fact inhibit authentic freedom. Whether in sickness or in health, living or dying, human nature strives for freedom.

The capacity for free choice entails the ego, which is the personal sense of liberty and the center of choice. The existence of the ego means that human nature has evolved beyond the archaic levels of the animal brain. Compared to that of animals, the human brain-mind system has achieved a high self-consciousness, including the personal knowledge of death. The unique aspect of human freedom is to experience self-consciousness in the face of death.

To understand the dynamics of the ego we follow Szondi's theory because he pioneered in establishing a synthesis for the schools of depth psychology (1956). Szondi's ego psychology is a comprehensive integration of heredity, instinctual drives, dreams, symbols, and faith. The ego is conceived in terms of choice behavior, and every decision reflects both inner and outer aspects. In the selection of a mate, an unconscious impulse is realized or consciously objectified in the other.

With the execution of the decision both subject and object converge in a reciprocal bond. The ego stands at the center of conscious and unconscious motivations and mediates the relationships.

Therefore, the ego is conceived dialectically and relationally. Viewing it either as subject or object, body or psyche, is to miss the essential wholeness. The ego is not conditioned exclusively by linear, causal processes but is more accurately understood as a complementary whole. Consequently, there are basically two kinds of choices made by humans. One affirms the essentially complementary nature of the organism and embraces antithetical strivings within oneself. The other type of choice acts out a single need, or a part, and becomes driven by contradictory and compulsive tendencies.

Accordingly, the ego may be considered in terms of two constitutive dimensions. One is the expansive, participatory aspect called the "p" dimension, and it consists of "the human need to make unconscious content conscious, and consequently to expand the ego-field" (Szondi 1956, 260). This expansive mode of thought informs both paranoia and authentic spiritual participation. Paranoia would be abnormal and spiritual presence normal. Whether the need for expansion results in normal or abnormal behavior depends upon how one participates in social and metaphysical reality. This expansive, participatory mode of the ego activates forms of the imagination, such as dreams and symbols.

The other dimension of the ego represents a controlling, practical mode of thought. Designated the "k" factor, this is "the human need to limit the boundless extended ego-field, to compress it" (Szondi 1956, 263). Since this need defends against unlimited, autistic, or impractical thought, it manifests individual identity, a perspectival ego, or the will. Its content is immanent consciousness, and its task is to adapt, make decisions, achieve mastery in the physical world. It is known as the "k" factor, because in its extreme abnormal state it becomes catatonia. (It is called "k," because the German spelling of catatonia is *katatonia*.) The catatonic personality is one who has achieved total control, total isolation, total impotence—in total defense against any higher forms of imagination, paranoia, autism, and authentic spiritual participation. In its normal phase, the perspectival ego satisfies the will or controlling "k" need.

These two modes of thought comprise the basic needs of the ego. They alternate in a dynamic rhythm, now one, now the other. The flow pattern is like that of blood pressure, a diastole and systole, expansion and contraction. In some cases, the dialectical flow can harden or split into inner conflicts. To illustrate these aspects some of the main characteristics are listed below (Szondi 1956, 276):

	Participatory Ego-"p"	Perspectival Ego-"k"
Functions:	Oneness and likeness with the other, doubling of the ego	Incorporation of the object, negation or destruction
Choice in love:	Projection	Introjection
Ideals:	Being	Having
Relationships:	Dual-union	Dominance-Submission
Social life:	Compassion, empathy	Compulsion, taboo
Character:	Introvert	Extrovert
Adaptation:	Participatory-inflative	Reality-testing
Worldview:	Spiritual	Material

In the face of death the perspectival ego attempts to secure control through the will, but it confronts the fact of having to die, which evokes anxiety. The will is powerless to remove anxiety as the basic symptom of death. As a result, in societies that encourage the power of having and the will cancer becomes pervasive. Clinically, the perspectival ego seeks control in terminal illness by creating stages, exerting denial, and erecting a taboo of silence around the dying patient. As subsequent chapters will demonstrate, only the participatory ego can make a meaningful adaptation to death.

When the participatory ego achieves high-level wholeness, by embracing the threat of death, it becomes the pontifical ego. Understood as the union of opposites, the pontifical ego (*Pontifex oppositorum*) manifests three clinical functions: participation, integration, and transcendence (Szondi 1956, 156). The pontifical ego embraces psychic antitheses and may be imagined as the axle of a wheel. The spokes are the antitheses and the revolving axle is the ego. It may also be imagined as a bridge, which spans a body of water, connecting this side with the other side. Since the pontifical ego represents a transcendent state of being, it cannot be affirmed directly by rational concepts but indirectly by negations, as is common in the mystical traditions of the world religions. Thus, Szondi describes the bridge by negation as

> ...neither spirit nor nature; it is the bridge between spirit and nature.
>
> The ego is neither object nor subject; it is the mediator between object and subject.
>
> The ego is neither waking nor dreaming; it is the bridge between waking and dreaming.
>
> The ego is neither this world nor the beyond; it is the bridge between this world and the beyond.

The notion of the pontifical or bridge-building ego (*Pontifex Ich*) is derived from the Latin terms for "bridge" (*Pons*) and for "making" (*facere*). Szondi retains the German word for ego (*Ich*) in order to emphasize that the participatory ideal does not contradict normal human capacities. However, in light of English usage, Szondi's concept is best expressed with the idea of self, because ego seems closer to the controlling, perspectival function.

Hence, pontifical selfhood fulfills the fundamental task of the human being, namely, the drive for oneness, likeness, and relatedness in social and metaphysical reality. Once primal participation is realized, even if only momentarily, integration and transcendence follow (Szondi 1956, 35). Integration means a unity of self and world, subject and object, and so forth. Transcendence means a projection of oneself onto a higher level, wherein one's power of being is exalted and the threat of death annulled.

The pontifical self is spaceless, timeless, and independent of causal law but informed by finality, which is the essential and complementary wholeness of reality. These characteristics are potentials in the unconscious. The worldview conforms to that in contemporary quantum-relativistic physics, wherein fundamental reality is conceived as pure energy without matter. By surpassing the three-dimensional world of ordinary life, pontifical selfhood actualizes a fourth dimension.

Since the ego is capable of finality, it cannot be located exhaustively in the body, brain, or mind. Its dynamic and potentially boundless relatedness permits translocal and transcausal exchanges, including clairvoyance and telepathy. In the fulfillment of the primal drive for participation, the self extends beyond itself in opposition to the body (Szondi 1956, 464). Thus, the exalted power of being actualizes transpersonal relatedness outside the body.

II. THE BRIDGE AS SYMBOL

In 1918 Carl Jung began to explore the centrality of symbolism in human experience. He sketched circular artistic forms as expressions of the inner life and gradually discovered the mandala as a primary archetype. Derived from the Sanskrit term for circle, a mandala is a work of art that corresponds to self-realization or individuation. Mandalas appear in dreams, mental disorders, and religious symbolism. They exhibit round, radial, or spherical patterns, and sometimes squares with a center, or even crosses. Mandalas are fixed by their respective religious and cultural traditions and transmitted consistently throughout the generations. Conceptually, mandalas conform to the quaternity, to which Jung assigns logical priority. A quaternity represents wholeness, and only four-fold statements are valid assertions of primal form.

Szondi acknowledges the mandala as a symbol of totality, but he gives priority to the bridge. The bridge is the preferred symbol, because wholeness is achieved by participation in a transcendent reality. Through projection, one goes beyond oneself to the distant shore, which is the other world and a transcendent dimension. The basic difference is that for Jung nothing ever exists outside the self, but for Szondi a genuinely spiritual reality lies beyond the self. Consequently, to exalt one's being is to "cross-over" to the distant shore and participate in fundamental, metaphysical reality.

To illustrate the pontifical ego Szondi draws upon the Hindu doctrine of the self (*Atman*), as portrayed in the Upanishads. Hinduism identifies the self with the Absolute (*Brahman*), which is the term for ultimate reality beyond subject and object. The Absolute is experienced as the fullness of being, consciousness, and joy. While Szondi appeals to the Upanishads, he goes beyond Hinduism, specifically, by emphasizing real otherness in the act of spiritual participation. Faith is an event of genuine dialogue and meeting (Szondi 1956, 519). In contrast, Hinduism claims that psychic opposites are completely dissolved in the ultimate state of self-realization. All conceptual thought, affective bonds, and unconscious dependence are abandoned. The attainment of primal being manifests an undifferentiated oneness. The Hindu concept presupposes the belief that consciousness is unlimited and omniscient, a point of view rejected by Szondi. For Szondi consciousness is limited to the immanent material world, and unconsciousness can never be removed, because it is the realm of the ancestors.

Nevertheless, Szondi recognizes that the Upanishads employ the bridge as a symbol of the self (1956, 114-115). One primary text is the Brhadaranyaka Upanishad (4. 4. 22.), which I cite using the Radhakrishnan translation (1953).

> Verily, he is the great unborn Self who is this (person) consisting of knowledge among the senses. In the space within the heart lies the controller of all, the lord of all, the ruler of all. He does not become greater by good works nor smaller by evil works. He is the bridge that serves as the boundary to keep the different worlds apart.

The Chandogya Upanishad presents the bridge symbol in two passages:

> Now the self is the bridge, the (separating) boundary for keeping these worlds apart. Over that bridge day and night do not cross, nor old age nor death, nor sorrow, nor well-doing nor ill-doing. All evils turn back from it for the Brahma-world is freed from evil (8. 4. 1.).
>
> Therefore, verily on crossing that bridge, if one is blind he becomes no longer blind, if wounded, he becomes no longer wounded, if afflicted, he becomes no longer afflicted. Therefore, verily, on crossing that bridge, night appears even as day for that Brahma-world is ever illumined (8. 4. 2.).

In each passage the phrase "Brahma-world" means the created, physical universe, which emanates from the Absolute.

The two Chandogya passages take the original Upanishadic image of the bridge as a separating-connecting function and expand it into a vision of immortality. This appears more clearly in the following two passages:

To him who is without parts, without activity, tranquil, irreproachable, without blemish, the highest bridge to immortality, like the fire with its fuel burnt (Svetesvatara 6. 19.).

He in whom the sky, the earth and the interspace are woven as also the mind along with all the vital breaths, know him alone as the one self. Dismiss other utterances. This is the bridge to immortality. May you be successful in crossing over to the farther shore of darkness (Mundaka 2. 2. 5-6.).

A similar motif appears in the Katha Upanishad (3. 2.): "That bridge for those who sacrifice, and which is the highest imperishable Brahman for those who wish to cross over to the farther fearless shore, that Naciket fire, may we master." This and the previous passages view time and eternity as separated by a gulf, which is represented by the river. This shore is the three dimensional, spatio-temporal, causal world, occupied by mortal human beings. The distant shore represents the fulfillment of selfhood, and the bridge is the disciplined process of self-realization. Thus, the bridge symbol fits the structure of the pontifical ego.

III. THE BRIDGE IN DEPTH PSYCHOLOGY

Even though Szondi made the bridge symbol central to his ego psychology, other depth psychologists have dealt with it to a certain extent. In two brief essays Sandor Ferenczi explores the psychoanalytic meaning of the bridge in dream and myth. He finds that the bridge symbol plays a striking role in the dreams of males and that it conveys images of sexuality, birth, and death. Through analysis of case materials Ferenczi believes that the bridge symbolizes the penis. The evidence for this interpretation is that male dreams display anxiety at or near a bridge and that this correlates with an inhibited ejaculation (Ferenczi 1921, 22). Collapse of a bridge signifies male impotence.

Ferenczi acknowledges that in society the bridge spans two separate landscapes. The bridge extends over flowing waters, which are dangerous and which symbolize the origins of life. Because of the primal imagery of water, the bridge represents the original union of mother and father in the act of copulation. Consequently, this shore means life as it is now, and the distant shore represents life that is not yet, namely, in the baby. Hence, the bridge is the male organ, passing over the uterine waters to a new life.

However, Ferenczi concedes that the bridge has other meanings as well. In his second essay he lists several meanings of the bridge symbol: (1) the male organ that unites parents in sexual intercourse and attaches itself to the child, so that it might not perish in the deep waters. (2) One is born into this world from the water; and the bridge connects this life and the unborn life. (3) The bridge spans death, which is a regression to the past, to maternal love, and to the uterine waters. (4) Finally, the bridge simply means crossing-over or changing conditions in one's life (Ferenczi 1922, 77).

Ferenczi's interpretation presupposes the psychoanalytic doctrine that sexual intercourse is a death experience. Ejaculation is a sacrifice and a narcissistic castration. Sexual union becomes paradise, and hell is the feeling of guilt and dread of punishment resulting from the sex act.

To challenge the psychoanalytic position I offer a teaching anecdote. In response to my discussion of the bridge symbol, during the spring semester of 1992, a female student wrote:

> During the last few months of my engagement, I would have strange dreams. I thought nothing of them until they were mentioned in this course. I had dreams of getting in a boat and rowing to an island, but never getting there. I also had very vivid dreams of a rope bridge. It was very high, connecting the woods to a mountain trail, and narrow. Everytime I had this dream, I would start across the bridge but never make it to the other side. Most of the time either the water below would rise up, and I would run back or the bridge would begin to rock back and forth so much that I had to cling for life out of fear of falling off into the waters below.

After receiving her paper, I spoke with her about her bridge dream, and she said that when she broke off the engagement, the dream ceased. I agreed with her decision and pointed out that the bridge appeared in the context of a mate selection and that falling off the bridge meant a wrong choice. Against Ferenczi's view the subject is female, and the context deals with destiny and not sexuality.

In Jungian psychology the bridge tends to be marginal, due to the priority of the mandala. However, Aniela Jaffè explains that the bridge symbolizes the connection between here and there, the present and the timeless, or the conscious and the unconscious (1963, 23). Frequently, the bridge symbol represents death and paranormal events. It is an archetype that shapes events, when the consciousness of participants is lowered or split. Jaffè cites an example of a woman who had decided to end an engagement.

> On a sparkling summer Sunday, I was walking with my mother across the Wettsteinbrücke at Basle to the other side of the Rhine. In her own inimitable way she was telling me stories of old Basle. I was listening enthralled. Suddenly I saw a broad beam of light falling from the sky, across the Rhine; my fiancé was coming towards me on it, and his eyes were fixed on me. I gazed at him in wonder, and heard the words: *That is your way.* The vision vanished and I heard my mother saying: "Whatever's the matter with you? I tell you stories and ask you questions and cannot get a word out of you. And you look dreadful—is anything the matter? You're as white as a sheet." But from that moment my way lay clear before me. Two years later we were married. There were hard times then and now, but always, when I nearly despaired, I saw the great beam of light and heard the words: *That is your way.* Even today I remember the very place where I had the vision (1963, 21).

This anecdote contains a three fold version of the bridge symbol. The woman is walking (1) on a physical bridge, when (2) "a great beam of light" bridges this world and the other world, and (3) she is absent-minded, which is an epileptiform phase that bridges consciousness and unconsciousness.

When applied to religious visions, the motif of the distant shore represents a transpersonal state, as Szondi's theory stipulates. The problem with the Jungian approach is that the other world is not reducible to the unconscious (Reimbold 1972, 73). Since in Jungian thought the bridge could refer to self-realization, then the flowing water rather than the distant shore should be interpreted as the unconscious. The bridge symbol has religious significance only if it designates a real self-transcendence.

The Szondian view of the bridge has been portrayed inadvertently in **The Bridge of San Louis Rey** by Thornton Wilder (1927). In fact, this novel bears a precise and uncanny resemblance to several central Szondian concepts. In the story a bridge has collapsed, and Brother Jupiter, the narrator, wonders whether the accident were by chance or by design. If the former, then the cause might be a latent factor in the victims themselves. One victim is a stutterer, who perceives people as egotistic and greedy, and who yearned for rebirth before her death. Another victim is the twin brother of a person who suffers fits of rage, and still another is a sufferer of outbursts of rage.

Wilder intuits a truth clinically documented by Szondi, that persons who carry epileptoid hereditary factors are vulnerable to accidents and to shock deaths. Brother Jupiter concludes that the collapse of the bridge had a reason, namely, to destroy the wicked and to save the good. He says that only love justifies human life and that love is the bridge between the living and the dead.

Finally, to illustrate the evocative power of the bridge symbol I recall how a student reacted to my discussion of it in the classroom on October 14, 1992. A student told me that in 1978 his father suffered a series of grand mal epileptic seizures, during which he had a vision of crossing a bridge to the distant shore. On the bridge the father heard a voice calling to him: "Come on over." He returned, however, to this shore and, sometime later, underwent surgery to remove a brain tumor.

Genetically, the father must be a carrier of threshold genes for epilepsy. One of his daughters is epileptic, and another is vulnerable to stuttering when removed from the enfolds of her community. The student himself suffers migraines, and he often dreams of grinding his teeth, breaking them, and spitting them out of his mouth. Since the common neurological explanation is that tumors often cause seizures in adults, in this case threshold genes have revealed the "Szondi Triad" in three siblings and the bridge symbol in a life-threatening situation of the father. Hence, epilepsy is genetically related to the symbolism of the bridge.

IV. ORIGIN OF THE CROSS-OVER ARCHETYPE

Although the bridge symbol appeared in the oldest Hindu Upanishads, written in the eighth century B.C.E., its religious significance actually extends far back into prehistoric times. In his classic essay on the bridge Frank Knight explains that all ancient peoples felt awe toward rivers and regarded them as obstacles in getting to the other side (1953, 848). Rivers were considered to be boundaries in the natural and divine scheme of the world. Erecting a bridge was believed to be an intrusion into the realm of the sacred; and so before building one, it was necessary to offer a sacrifice in appeasement of the river deity. Sacrifices at the river were a foundational ritual and basic to cultural and religious development.

Making sacrifices prior to bridge-building entails a primal mystique of water, a fact confirmed by archeology, particularly in Northwestern Europe (Hutton 1991, 59, 109-110, 184-187, 210-230). People of the Bronze Age (2200-1000 B.C.E.) in the British Isles threw precious objects as sacrifices into rivers, pools, or bogs. The practice surely precedes the Bronze Age, because many of the objects were Neolithic flints, weapons, and ornaments. Within England the rivers chosen for this custom all flow to the East. For example, the Thames River has skulls and stripped skeletons, suggesting the Neolithic practice of stripping flesh from corpses. Rivers flowing in other directions have been dredged, but no precious sacrificial objects have been found.

An inventory of these river objects discloses a pattern. Shields and vessels were deposited in bogs and pools, but swords were cast into rivers. The swords were always broken before being thrown away. In contrast, on the continent of Europe swords were buried in the ground and not cast into the water. Thus, the British practice implies a sacrificial offering to the sacred waters, and the sacredness of water survives in the term "latis" which means "pool-goddess." The term was used for place names in Northern England, during the Roman period (43-410 C.E.).

Of the objects dredged from British rivers are many forms of the Celtic cross, consisting of a wheel encircling a cross and comprising a four-spoked wheel. The Celtic cross is also prominent in Scandinavian rock art, where it is carried by boats, ships, carts, or chariots. Even some of the British and Scandinavian tombs were constructed in the shape of boats or timber canoes. For example, the Suffolk coast of England was the site of large ship burials, and in Scandinavian societies boats carrying the dead were set adrift or burned at sea.

Jungians would interpret the Celtic cross as a mandala, but this would be misleading for two reasons. First, there is no evidence that the Celtic cross represents self-realization or the union of consciousness and unconsciousness. Second, Bronze Age tombs and monuments are aligned with the sky, with the movement of the sun and the succession of the seasons. This fact suggests that the Celtic cross symbolizes the crossing of the sun or the turning of the heavens. The image of the cross as a wheel is reinforced by its relation with carts and chariots in rock art. Thus, no evidence obtains for linking the crossing of the sun with the hero myth, as Jung claims.

Throwing a Celtic cross into a river or emblazoning it in a tomb suggests that the crossing of the sun was linked to death. Death was represented by a boat moving across the waters or a cart making a journey. Either motif coincided with the crossing pattern of the sun. Since the rivers containing crosses flow to the East, from where the sun rises in the morning, then death would imply a turning toward the source of light. In any case, such an interpretation would come from a projection by peoples participating in rituals of death.

This possibility is supported by an extraordinary archeological finding. Among the tombs of Neolithic Ireland (3200-2200 B.C.E.) that of Knowth's Passage features an entrance, above which is a small opening. The body was inserted, head first, into the entrance, and its face turned toward the small opening above the entrance. We are naturally inclined to ask why a separate opening exists above the entrance. Why not raise the entrance? The question may be answered by performing a simple experiment. If one were to crawl into the tomb and look toward the opening, one would realize that only on one day of the year sunlight would penetrate the opening and fill the chamber with a glowing red spiral. That time is the dawn of the winter solstice. As explained by the principal investigator, the small opening allowed the sun to enter and radiate the face of the deceased, because "the beautiful appearance of the rising solstice sun was not intended for the rituals of the living. It was for the dead" (Hutton 1991, 59).

The tomb was made so that only on the day of the winter solstice the rays of the sun became a bridge, on which the soul of the deceased crossed over the sky to a new life. The eerie red glow in the tomb transfigured death into a radiant state. Thus, a radiant vision of death joined the primal cross-over pattern of the sun, as an expansion of the burial ritual. Out of the cross-over motif came the Celtic cross, boats, ships, carts, and chariots as symbols of death.

This interpretation helps explain why sacrificial objects were only thrown into British rivers flowing east. Water that flowed to the horizon where the sun rises is sacred, and a sacrifice to the river deity facilitates new life. Rivers flowing to the west are not sacred, because the western horizon is where the sun sets. This insight gave rise to the symbol of the West as the land of death, where the sun descends to journey through the underworld. The underworld journey complements the crossing of the sun in the day and makes a vast cosmic wheel, so that in life and death the world turns.

V. ANCESTRAL CROSS-OVER PATTERN

Archeological evidence for an archaic cross-over motif also comes from Australian Aboriginal culture, which sustained a continuous history from about three million to 10,000 years ago. Approximately, 400,000 years ago Aboriginal ancestors appeared on the Australian continent, having evolved from *Homo Erectus* or so-called Java man, who dates from about one million years ago. New archeological evidence demonstrates a connection between Java man of Indonesia and the Australian Aborigines. They share a common skeletal type, namely, that of large robust faces, thick bones, and curved eyes (Flood 1988, 55-60, 70-73). Waves of Java man emigrated to Australia about 400,000 years ago where later they evolved into *Homo Sapiens* or the modern human race. The dating of 400,000 years derives from the use of mitochondrial DNA in the mapping of the human family tree. Unlike nuclear DNA, mitochondrial DNA is transmitted only by the mother, so that its genes are not shuffled and recombined. It evolves ten times faster than nuclear DNA. The traditional date of the origin of *Homo Sapiens*, inferred from nuclear DNA, had been 100,000 years ago. Thus, mitochondrial DNA pushes human origins further back and links them to the cross-over archetype.

Asian ancestors of the Aborigines emigrated to Australia, when sea levels were low and the ice age had laid down continuous links between the Northern Australian landmass and that of Southeastern Asia, where Java man lived. The people emigrated by walking the ice-bridges and by making rustic crafts to cross the waters. The crafts were constructed of logs, bamboo, and cords, which were available in Southeast Asia. Once the people had crossed over to Australia, their crafts were so damaged that they could not return. They remained, settled Australia, and evolved into the modern human race without competition from other species.

The emigration has been preserved in narrative form through the oral tradition. Central to the Aboriginal tradition is the mythology of the

Dreamtime, which is the time when the ancestors came across the sea in canoes. One person recalls

> That my own people, the Riratjingu, are descended from the great Djankawu who came from the island of Baralku far across the sea. Our spirits return to Baralku when we die. Djankawu came in his canoe with his two sisters, following the morning star which guided them to the shores of Yelangbara on the eastern coast of Arnhem Land. They walked far across the country following the rain clouds (Marika 1980, 5).

The Dreamtime is occupied by the Spirit Ancestors, who give life and receive the dead. One of the Spirit Ancestors is the giant Rainbow Serpent who, the informant continues,

> ...emerged from beneath the earth and as she moved, winding from side to side, she forced her way through the soil and rocks, making the great rivers flow in her path, and carving through mountains she made the gorges of northern Australia. From the Rainbow Serpent sprang many tribes, and tales about her are told all over Arnhem Land....

The symbol of the Rainbow Serpent belongs to the mythologies of rains and floods, motifs that reflect ecological conditions following the end of the last ice age. At that time temperatures rose, drying up the valleys, melting the ice bridges at the edge of the continental shelf, and flooding the land. Symbolizing these elemental forces, the mythic Rainbow Serpent emerged about 9000 years ago, making it one of the oldest and continuous figures in the world. Since it links the Dreamtime of the Spirit Ancestors to the historical time of the Aboriginal descendants, it functioned as a bridge symbol.

From all of this archeological evidence I infer the existence of an archaic cross-over archetype. The cross-over is just as universal as the Creation myths (Lauf 1980, 83). Both the cross-over and Creation presuppose a separation of this world and the beyond as well as the elements of air, earth, fire, and water. These are shock symbols, applicable to death and to creation. However, the cross-over archetype stands at the origins of human culture, as the Australian Aborigines demonstrate. With reference to the British and Scandinavian materials, cited in section four, tombs and monuments appeared between the end of the ice age, when the British Isles broke away from Europe, and the classical civilizations of Mesopotamia and Egypt. British prehistory has the cross-over motif in the adoration of the sun, burial of the dead, and the sanctity of water.

The relationship between the sun, the wheel, and the dead bears upon the theme of this book. Facing a burial chamber toward the sun of the winter solstice, as at Knowth's Passage, radiates the dead and presumes that the soul of the deceased will travel across the sky on the rays of the sun to a new life. Envisioning the dead in terms of the solar cycle is a forthright attempt to cope with the threat of death; for circular rotation is a symbolization of a shock event.

VI. THE BRIDGE IN FOUNDATION MYTH

When the cross-over archetype takes shape as a bridge, the symbol functions as a foundation myth of various cultures. One example is the Creation story of Imperial Japan called *Kojiki*. It narrates the creation of the *Kami* which are sacred forces that pervade nature in mystery and awe. Of the *Kami* two are the primal man (*Izanagi*) and primal woman (*Izanami*). Chapter three tells how they solidify the land by creating Onogoro island.

> Thereupon, the two deities stood on the Heavenly Floating Bridge and, lowering the jeweled spear, stirred with it. They stirred the brine with a churning-churning sound, and when they lifted up [the spear] again, the brine dripping down from the tip of the spear piled up and became an island, this was the island Onogoro (Earhart 1974, 15).

The primal pair descend on the bridge from the heavens to the island, where they make a large palace and heavenly pillar. *Izanami* and *Izanagi* marry and copulate, at first unsuccessfully but later successfully. When *Izanami* gives birth to fire, she is fatally burned, and she descends to the underworld. Her husband follows her into the underworld and attempts to restore her to life. He fails and ascends to the surface, where 'he purifies himself and resumes procreation. The story culminates in the creation of the ancestral gods and the enthronement of *Amaterasu*, Sun Goddess and ancestor of the emperor.

The Japanese Creation Narrative does not support the psychoanalytic interpretation of the bridge. The primal man and woman do not copulate on the bridge but in the social world, after descending from the bridge. Death is not associated with the bridge but with the making of fire. Since the ancestors descend from heaven on the bridge, it provides a means of reciprocal participation between them and their descendants. In modern Japan bridges link the sacred world of the Shinto shrines and the profane world.

As a part of foundation mythology, the bridge may shape beliefs concerning the end of the world. For example, among the Winnebago Tribe of Native Americans, the dying receive instruction on how to travel the road to the land of the dead. One must have the sacred pipe and tobacco, fire and food, as well as a war club to hit objects on the road. One arrives at a round lodge and meets an old woman; she boils rice and gives it to the deceased, who eats it and gets a headache.

> Then she will break open your skull and take out your brains and you will forget all about your people on earth and where you come from. You will not worry about your relatives. You will become like a holy spirit.
>
> You are to take the four steps because the road will fork there. All your relatives (who died before you) will be there. As you journey on you will come to a fire running across the earth from one end to the other. There will be a bridge across it but it will be difficult to cross because it is continually swinging. However, you will be able to cross it safely, for you have all the guides about whom the warriors spoke to you. They will take you over and take care of you.
>
> Well, we have told you a good road (to take). If anyone tells a falsehood in speaking of the spirit-road, you will fall off the bridge and be burned. However (you need not worry) for you will pass over safely. As you proceed from that place the spirits will come to meet you and take you to the village where the chief lives (Radin 1970, 96).

The deceased gives tobacco to the chief, after which he or she enters a large lodge and greets the ancestors.

Finally, Germanic mythology has the *Bifrost* bridge, which is a quivering rainbow, burning with fire, linking heaven and earth and allowing the gods to travel over it. In Old Norse literature, the *Gjallar* bridge evolved with the vision literature of Europe, where in the vision of Olav Asteson, it is "'so high up in the air' decked with red-gold and gold pinnacles. A serpent, a dog, and a bull were there 'fierce and wroth' to prevent passing over" (Patch 1980, 122). This theme is a part of the Medieval European notion of the bridge of danger ("Brig o' Dread") and bridge of anxiety (*"Pont qui Tremble"*).

VII. THE ESCHATOLOGICAL BRIDGE

When the bridge motif features danger and obstacles, it takes another function, an eschatological symbol of conscience and selfhood at the end of the world. Emphasis on conscience in the eschatological bridge became clear during the transition from the Old Iranian religion to Zoroastrianism. The Old Iranian heritage developed between 5000 and 2000 B.C.E., and it included creation narratives of the separation of heaven and earth, the intermediate world, and the ·Chinvat crossing (Gnoli 1989, 125). The Chinvat crossing was probably "a ford over an underground river, guarded by supernatural dogs" (Boyce 1990, 10). When reaching the Chinvat crossing, the male met his soul in the form of a beautiful girl. The Chinvat crossing was the passage of the deceased to the Kingdom of the Dead, ruled by Yima, the first king and the first man to die. Originally, only heroic persons crossed Chinvat and entered Yima's Kingdom. If worshipped properly, they would protect their descendants. As hope in paradise gradually became more general, Chinvat crossing became Chinvat Bridge, the link between heaven and earth.

The Old Iranian vision of the bridge entered Hinduism during the Vedic period, when the Persian warrior tribes invaded India beginning about 1500 B.C.E. and ending about the time the Upanishads were being compiled. Thus, the Upanishadic descriptions of the bridge, discussed in section two, reflected the Iranian heritage.

However, the Chinvat Bridge attained its clearest and most distinct form in Zoroastrianism, particularly in the sayings of the prophet Zoroaster called Gathas and in the liturgy or Yasna. These materials portray the prophet guiding the good one over the Chinvat Bridge to Paradise. The oldest text is Yasna 46:10, and for citations of this and subsequent passages I use the new translations by Mary Boyce (1990, 39, 42-43, 80-83):

> Whosoever, Lord, man or woman, will grant me those things
> thou knowest best for life—recompense for truth, power with
> good purpose—and those whom I shall bring to your worship,
> with all these I cross over the Chinvat Bridge (Yas. 46:10).
>
> Thus the Inner Self of the wicked man destroys for him the
> reality of the straight way. His soul shall surely vex him at the
> Chinvat Bridge, for he has strayed from the path of truth by his
> acts and (the words) of his tongue (Yas. 51:13).

In this second passage the soul is called *daena*, and it appears along side
the bridge, preventing the wicked from crossing. One is then damned.
Here the term *daena* means religion and the inner self, as clarified in
Yasna 31:20: "...O wicked ones, your inner self shall lead you by her
actions."

Subsequent texts have elaborated the images of *daena* and the bridge.
In the Vendidad, the Younger Avestan writings from the Parthian period
(141 B.C.E.-224 C.E.), it is stated:

> It (the soul) goes along the paths created by time for both the
> wicked and the just, to the Mazda-created Chinvat Bridge....
> There comes that beautiful one, strong, fair of form,
> accompanied by the two dogs.... She comes over high Hara
> [mountain], she takes the souls of the just over the Chinvat
> Bridge, to the rampart of the invisible yazatas (Vd. 19:29-30).

In Zoroastrianism the dog mediates the human and spiritual worlds.
This role of the dog survives from the old Indo-Iranian religion, where
dogs are the messengers of Yima. The soul, whom the two dogs
accompany, is described even further in the Hadhokht Nask text:

> As that wind blows on him, his own Daena appears in the form
> of a maiden, beautiful, queenly, white-armed,...in shape as
> beautiful as the most beautiful of creatures. Then the soul of the
> just man said to her, inquiring: "What girl are you, the most
> beautiful in form of all girls that I have ever seen?" Then his
> own Daena answered him: "Truly, youth of good thoughts,
> good words, good acts, good inner self (daena), I am your very
> own Daena." (2. 24-26).

In Zoroastrian doctrine the soul lingers near the corpse three days after death. At dawn of the fourth day the soul ascends by the light of the sun to the Chinvat Bridge. The just soul meets the beautiful girl, aged 15, who comprises one's good thoughts, words, and actions in one's own life. The bridge is wide, and she leads the soul across to Paradise. With the death of the unjust person, the soul

> weeps, saying: "Whither shall I go and whom shall I now take as refuge?" And it sees with its eyes, during those three days and nights, all the sins and wickedness which it has done in the world. On the fourth day the demon Vizarsh comes and binds the wicked man's soul in the harshest way, and,...leads it to the Chinvat Bridge.
>
> And the wicked person's soul will cry out with loud lamentations and will weep and utter many pleas, entreatingly, and make many desperate struggles in vain. And since his struggles and entreaties are of no avail at all, and no good being nor yet devil comes to his aid, the demon Vizarsh drags him evilly to...hell. And then a girl approaches, not like other girls. And the wicked man's soul says to that hideous girl: "Who are you, than whom I have never seen a girl more hideous and hateful?" And answering him she says: "I am no girl, but I am your own acts, O hateful one of bad thought, bad word, bad act, bad inner self" (Menog i Khrad, 2:159-171).

Finally, the mature conception of the Chinvat Bridge comes in the ninth century C.E. text, Dadestan i denig, question 20:3-7:

> The [Chinvat] Bridge is like a sword..., one of whose surfaces is broad, one narrow and sharp. With its broad side, it is so ample that it is twenty-seven poles wide; with its sharp side, it is so constructed that it is as narrow as a razor's edge. When the souls of the just and the wicked arrive, it turns on that side which is required for them, through the great glory of the Creation,...it becomes a broad crossing for the just..., for the wicked it becomes a narrow crossing, just like a razor's edge. The soul of a just person crosses the Bridge, and its way is pleasantness. When that of a wicked person sets foot on the

Bridge, because of the...sharpness it falls from the middle of the Bridge and tumbles down.

Variations of the Chinvat Bridge survive in other religious traditions. Islamic eschatology envisions, at the end of time, total destruction of the world, followed by resurrection and the last judgment. In the judgment each person's deeds are weighed, and he or she is assigned to a particular group, depending on one's evaluation. Both the good and the bad cross over the bridge (*al-Sirat*) in order to verify their judgment. The bridge is not a test, since the judgment has been completed. In Islamic theology "the *sirāt* is finer than a hair and sharper than a sword; on its edges are metal hooks that grab onto one. If a person falls it involves a 3000 year journey—1000 climbing back up, another 1000 trying to travel along the bridge, and again another falling down" (cited in Smith and Haddad 1981, 215). The destination of the good is the Garden and that of the bad the Fire.

A more condensed version of the bridge entered Hasidic Judaism, specifically, in the teachings of Rabbi Nachman of Bratslav, who lived in the late eighteenth and early nineteenth centuries C.E.. He held a gloomy, pessimistic worldview, and he encouraged his disciples to live by faith, hope, and joy. He said: "The entire world is a very narrow bridge; the main thing is to have no fear" (Witztum, et. al., 1990, 125).

VIII. CONSCIENCE, BRIDGE, AND SELFHOOD

The foregoing survey gives evidence of the bridge as a basic symbol in some of the major religions of the world. The classical form originated in Old Iranian religion, and from there passed into Hinduism and Zoroastrianism. The Zoroastrian version survived in Islam and Judaism. The Christian variant will be discussed in chapter eight. After splitting off from Hinduism, Buddhism refined the vision of the distant shore into a symbol of enlightenment. It imagined the life process as the flow of a wide river and its teaching as a crossing over the waters on a craft. In modern Japanese Buddhism the vision of the distant shore is represented in the bridges, which are common to Zen gardens. The Zen master Hakuin painted a famous painting of "Blind Men Crossing a Bridge" to express the danger of life's passage.

To ground the bridge symbol in the psychology of death it is necessary to analyze the implied psychodynamics, using the Chinvat

Bridge as the model. The central issue is the meaning of the *daena*, which meets the soul of the deceased on the bridge.

Psychoanalysis would interpret the *daena* as the mother figure for the deceased male or the father figure for the deceased female. The reason for this view is that later Zoroastrian texts compare death with birth. When the soul lingers near the corpse three days after death, and is buffeted by the wind, then this is the same as labor prior to delivery (Molé 1960, 175). Thus, the female *daena* on the bridge is the mother who delivers a new birth to the deceased male. This psychoanalytic argument reduces the birth-death relation to one of identity.

However, the psychoanalytic view is contradicted by the fact that the *daena* or inner self is created by God from the beginning as announced in Yasna 39:11:

Since, O Mazda, Thou didst fashion for us in the beginning, by the thought, creatures and inner selves and intentions, since Thou didst create corporeal life, and acts and words through which he who has free will expresses choices....

The inherent capacity for free choice is guided by ancestral rituals, specifically, initiation at age 15. The fact that the *daena* is a 15 year old presupposes the normative value of initiation. In light of the Gathas *daena* means the religion of Zoroaster, accomplished properly by the initiation, and which shapes one's life after death (Molé 1960, 170). The *daena* is the religious model that the 15 year old assimilates at initiation.

The Jungian interpretation comes from Henry Corbin, who says that

Daena is, in fact, the feminine Angel who typifies the transcendent or celestial "I;" she appears to the soul at the dawn following the third night after its departure from this world; she is its Glory and its Destiny, its *Aean*. The meaning...is that the substance of the celestial "I" or Resurrection Body is engendered and formed from the celestial Earth....(1977, 15)

Corbin clarifies the phrase "Glory and its Destiny" with two Greek terms: *Doxa* and *Tyche*, which mean "glory" and "chance," respectively. As the "light of Glory," the *daena* is the transfigured power of the soul, which is not sensory but an inner visionary ability. Corbin stipulates that the *daena* is "the vision of the celestial world as it is *lived*, that is, as religion and professed faith in essential individuality" (1977, 42). The *daena* is a guardian angel, judge, or soul on the way to fulfillment, and the Chinvat Bridge is a projection of the process of completion. With respect to Jungian psychology, the *daena* is the anima, or soul of the male represented by a female archetype, and the bridge is the process of self-realization or individuation.

Corbin's profound and elegant definition clearly brings out the essential, mystical aspect of the *daena*. However, the embodiment of the three-fold ethic in the *daena* (good thought, word, and deed) rejects the quaternity and suggests the conquest and restitution of evil (bad thought, word, and deed). The *daena* manifests the conscience of the person who has enacted the ethic since initiation (Molé 1960, 163-166). Consequently, the *daena* reveals a pattern of destiny which, as it plays out in the life of a person, is closer to a necessity than to chance. One's destiny necessitates the kind of *daena* revealed on the Chinvat Bridge.

The notions of conscience and destiny go beyond Jung to Szondi, from whose perspective the Chinvat Bridge is the pontifical self. Since the bridge spans this shore and the distant shore, life and death, good and evil, male and female, then it symbolizes the union of psychic antitheses. Szondi contends that the crucial condition for achieving a full selfhood is the restitution of evil, which brings liberation and wholeness. Restitution of evil is his basic definition of conscience, and it obtains when one's evil nature, one's Cain intent, is transferred onto God, who alone ultimately atones for all evil. Projection of oneself onto God makes possible participation in ultimate spiritual reality (Szondi 1973, 148-149). Thus, the *daena* is conscience in the sense that its ethical function of atonement brings about the pontifical phases of participation, integration, and transcendence. Only through a conscientious faith can human nature be fulfilled, and the love of God revealed.

CHAPTER FOUR:
DREAMS AND VISIONS OF DEATH

I. PARTICIPATORY DREAMWORK

In this and the following two chapters the relation between death and participatory selfhood is explored in terms of dreams and visions. Since terminal illness and bereavement usually come under medical management, dreams and visions are often dismissed by health-care givers as hallucinations or delusions. Such interpretations are philosophical judgments that exceed the boundaries of medicine and need to be challenged.

To clarify these issues the respective terms should be defined. Hallucinations are a discharge of sensory material from within the central nervous system that does not cohere with the objective socio-physical environment. One who hallucinates seems confused and incoherent. Hallucinations may be caused by bodily traumas, high fever, poison, or medications. The basic characteristic of hallucinations is that they do not change the person's life or attitude. One remains the same before and after hallucinating, namely, with impaired reality testing.

Delusion is similar to hallucination, except that it falsifies reality, and is driven by internal disturbances and defective relatedness. Whereas hallucination is a distortion of perception, delusion is an erroneous view of the world that substitutes for genuine participation (Szondi 1956, 413, 451). One who is deluded desires to relate socially and metaphysically but cannot. Instead one surrenders to substitute forms of satisfaction determined by a specific ego phase, such as projection or inflation. Whatever the mode, one needs delusion to cope with a basic insecurity, fear of aloneness, and anxiety of death.

A vision is an experience in which symbolic content enters the mind from an outside source, whether unconscious or transcendent. The most distinctive traits are a mandate, such as a summons or a calling, and, consequently, profound changes in the personality (Benz 1968, 10-11). The mandate is self-evident and self-authenticating. To a certain extent, a vision resembles a dream; however, the dream presents indirect or symbolic forms that require interpretation.

Generally, in the history of religions little dreams are distinguished from big dreams. The former express content entirely within the dreamer's personal experience, but the latter are exclusively symbolic, containing ancestral models and/or archetypes from within traditional religions and mythologies. Big dreams are like visions, and, in the history of religions, they are paired with each other. However, dreams come during sleep while visions could appear in sleep, in waking consciousness, or upon awakening. Furthermore, a vision could bring a separation from the body, otherworld journey, and ecstasy. Thus, the vision would exemplify an expansive, participatory mode of thought in opposition to the body, as Szondi would say.

The visionary is grasped by ultimate reality, which makes the mandate compelling. Visionary material may be imaginal, visual, or auditory. Historically, mystics have tried to go beyond sensory visions to image-less states of pure being or nothingness. Since some visions impart pure experience, it is difficult to define them exclusively as projections of the unconscious. When symbolism is present, surely the unconscious plays some role in the vision; and the law of participation, formulated by Szondi, provides a comprehensive framework. When the visionary is grasped by ultimate reality, he or she is simultaneously driven toward participation in fundamental reality. Sensory modes, even conscious and unconscious, may be regarded as phases along the way to pontifical selfhood and its functional characteristics of participation, integration, and transcendence.

Closely related to the vision is the apparition, defined as a spontaneous breakthrough from a transpersonal source into the natural world, while the latter remains unchanged and correlated with personal consciousness (Dinzelbacher 1978, 117). When beholding an apparition, one does not separate from the body. An apparition resembles a vision in the sense that it may come to waking consciousness and deliver a mandate. However, unlike the vision, an apparition may be seen by more than one person and have an objective quality, spatial form, or mass without matter. An apparition may move, vibrate, or radiate energy in morphic fields. Like the dream and vision, an apparition conforms to the law of participation and presents a narrative framework as complementary to organic and interpersonal dimensions. Apparition, dream, and vision all bear co-acting transpersonal and unconscious functions as well.

Furthermore, apparition, dream, and vision may involve a synchronicity, a phenomenon emphasized by Jungian psychology. Jung defines a synchronicity as a meaningful coincidence of two or more psychic or physical events, which are separated in space and cannot be explained by causal interaction (1960, 441). The simultaneous and meaningful coming together of distant events is governed by an archetype. Under the impact of synchronicity, the psyche is relativized. The three dimensional, spatio-temporal, causal world is temporarily suspended, as the collective unconscious realizes a purposive unity. Since the Jungian definition of the psyche is deficient, with respect to the family, it is necessary to add that the ancestry may also inform a synchronicity. Both ancestral and archetypal forms share translocal and transcausal exchanges within the unconscious.

All of the foregoing phenomena may be viewed in terms of Szondi's participatory theory of dreams. Szondi defines the dream as a nocturnal search for a oneness, likeness, and relatedness between waking consciousness or foreground and the hidden, unconscious background (1956, 466). Achieving such a unity obtains an "autogenic participation." The uniqueness of this participation is that the dream exceeds the boundaries of the spatio-temporal, causal world, penetrating the "beyond" in the sense of an unconscious "split-off" phase. Such a "split-off" phase, however, is not delusory but participatory.

To a certain extent, Szondi's dream theory resembles Jung's. Jung grounds his dream theory in the concept of compensation. The dream compensates the perspective of consciousness. When the consciousness becomes too one-sided, the dream automatically compensates through the elemental forces of the archetypes. Compensation compares to the automatic swinging of a pendulum or to the self-regulating forces of nature. Just as nature balances itself, so does the dream. Dreaming belongs to nature; it is trustworthy and not deceitful.

Szondi founds his theory upon the concept of complementarity. He would agree with Freud that dreams reflect causes from the past and with Jung that they forecast the future or manifest finality, but he would contend that the motor force of dreaming is the primal drive for participation. The complementary parts of the dream are the waking or foreground self (*Vorder-Ich*) and the latent, hidden, or background self (*Hinter-Ich*), which contains repressed, instinctual drives and hereditary material. Each self complements the other, and each revolves with the other. These rotating phases are consistent with the functions of threshold genes and with dominance variability.

Dreams may be analyzed in terms of four dramatic phases (Szondi 1956, 487-489). (1) The waking ego prepares for a journey by exploring various existential possibilities. This preparation takes place at the beginning of the dream cycle. (2) The waking ego surpasses a threshold, becoming hypnagogic, and descends into a deeper, symbolic background. As an example, one goes through a tunnel or across a bridge; or one sinks into a depth or into a whirlpool. (3) At a profound level awareness becomes purely symbolic; this is the dream world, as such. The waking ego withdraws from the scene, becomes a passive spectator, and watches the action unfold on the stage; out of the unconscious, the personal, familial, and/or collective figures step forth. Frequently, ancestral models are presented, so that one receives a freedom of choice and is able to choose more than one existential possibility. (4) Finally, the self becomes hypnopompic. The waking ego comes out from the background into center stage, and then the dreamer awakens. Symbolically, one goes up a staircase, or returns from a trip to one's family or place of work.

By describing these phases dramatically, as though they were four acts of a play, Szondi produces a narrative structure. Within the dramatic narrative the second and fourth phases are pivotal; for they signify two thresholds, respectively, in which the waking ego transcends itself. Whereas in Jung's theory such phases would only compensate for the extremes of consciousness, in Szondi's a basic decision-making role of the dream is uncovered. Choices are posed with respect to existential possibilities which the dreamer may be affirming and those which may be hidden or repressed. Since dreamers often neglect or forget material from the threshold phases, dream interpretation frequently fails to clarify the decision-making possibilities of the dream.

The narrative structure of Szondi's theory also complements the internal rhythms of creativity that emerge in the dream stages of sleep. It is well-known that sleep goes through ninety minute cycles of the night. Expressed by rapid-eye movements, dreaming may be as short as ten minutes or as long as one or two hours. Unlike deep sleep which lacks rapid-eye movements, dreaming is one form of seizure activity, as Frederic Myers knew so long ago. Dreaming is, according to the new scientific studies, "the conscious experience of a normal nocturnal brain seizure which helps the brain avoid the excessive excitability that plagues epilepsy victims even during the waking state" (Hobson 1988, 176). This relationship with epilepsy reveals alternating phases of neural activities, one dominant and one recessive. These patterns demonstrate that the brain sustains wave-like, undulating rhythms in itself. Dreaming takes place when the paroxysmal, reticular neurons dominate and escape the inhibitory aminergic neurons (ibid, 184). Switching on and off the polar paroxysmal and inhibitory functions starts in the brain stem and is mediated by a functional disinhibition. Thus, every dreamer is a latent epileptic.

The imagery of dream sleep is volitional, creative, and adaptive. Dreaming discharges intense emotion, which is channelled by instinctual drives and genetic information encoded in the animal brain. These functional aspects are consolidated by symbolism, through which the primal drive for participation achieves a unity of self. Dreams, visions, and apparitions deliver a narrative framework to the drive for participation, even in the face of death.

II. DREAMS AND TERMINAL CANCER

According to classical psychoanalytic doctrine, dreams of the dying tend to be simple fulfillments of childhood desires, based upon regression, and aimed toward a denial of death. This approach presupposes Freud's influential opinion that the unconscious lacks knowledge of death and has neither contradiction nor negation (S.E. XIV, 1957a, 296). For Freud the unconscious believes in its own immortality. In contrast, subsequent clinical work has revealed that regressive wish-fulfilling dreams exist independently of a denial of death and belief in immortality (Norton 1963). Phases of denial, depression, and heightened narcissism belong to the grieving process, which includes unconscious and/or conscious knowledge of death.

More recently, dreams of fourteen terminally ill cancer patients were compared with those of healthy, elderly persons. Despite a conscious denial of death, the dreams of the cancer patients revealed an unconscious knowledge of death (Coolidge and Fish 1983-1984). Along with themes of death, the dreams of the cancer patients expressed fear and loneliness, indicating the discharge of emotion.

Emotions relate to aggression, which, the authors find, occurs in 50% of the dreams of cancer patients. They theorize that the projection of aggression in dreams reflects the dreamer's attitude toward dying. When the dreamer is the object, then death is the aggressor; but when the dreamer is the subject, then aggression displaces anger or rage against death by falling onto other characters. Other persons in the dream are usually members of one's own family. Projecting death onto another character implies the dreamer's own ambivalence toward dying.

The authors conclude that death dreams are attempts to integrate the unconscious knowledge of death with consciousness. This conclusion is sound, and it reveals the knowledge of death to be a threshold function. The dreams discharge paroxysmal aggression in an attempt to bring the unconscious fear and loneliness in the face of one's death across the threshold of consciousness.

In another study Charles Garfield reports his work with 215 terminal cancer patients over a three year span. He discovers his patients to have ambivalence, increasing weakness, and an "altered state of consciousness" just before death. The idea of "altered state" is not defined, but it represents the time when dreams and visions are active. Garfield describes the following symbolic patterns of dreams and visions: (1) real and radiant encounters of light, celestial music, deceased and religious figures; (2) clear and demonic, nightmarish imagery; (3) alternating blissful and terrifying dream-like images; and (4) the void and/or the tunnel (1979, 54).

Garfield mentions that his patients suffer severe chemo-therapeutic and radiological toxins, but he does not explain how these correlate with the dreams and visions. Neither he nor the authors cited above discuss medical factors, such as fever, pain, or medications as variables. Are the dreams and visions products of or defenses against pain? In the absence of an answer in their studies, I would go on and say no, because dreams and visions tend to diminish pain. The reason is that the pain threshold is not reducible to physical sensations but varies with respect to situational factors and religious or cultural meaning (Blumer 1975, 871-872).

In summary, these studies of cancer patients' dreams yield significant conclusions: (1) The intent of death dreams and visions is to integrate the foreground and background selves with knowledge of impending death. (2) Radiance and creativity signify integration. (3) Demonic and threatening images represent a failure to achieve integration, a failure to surpass the threshold of consciousness, by not resolving conflict, ambivalence, or hostility. (4) The void and tunnel suggest lack of integration due to helplessness, despair, or depression.

III. ARCHETYPAL DEATH VISIONS

Jung emphasizes that the symptoms of dying operate in the unconscious long before death and that the purpose of the psyche is to prepare consciousness for impending death through dreams and visions (1960, 411). Jung's view opposes Freud's belief that the unconscious lacks a knowledge of death. Jung maintains that the unconscious is both aware of death and a life after death.

When a natural terminal process sets in, the unconscious symbolizes death as a journey. Aniela Jaffè explains that her father

> had been an invalid for a long time as the result of an accident. When at last the time came for him to die, he said to my dear mother and to relatives at midday that he was going home by the night train at half-past-twelve. And he died to the very minute....(1963, 413)

She goes on to say the image of farewell is related to that of the journey and that it usually brings a melancholic serenity to the survivors. She illustrates with a dream of the deceased in a forest:

> I called out a cheerful greeting to him. My brother-in-law smiled and waved back, but when we were about ten yards from each other, he turned down another path, smiled at me again and once more waved his hand. As I had not seen my brother-in-law for years, I was quite taken aback and woke up. The dream was so vivid that I lay awake for hours thinking about it. On the following day I received, to my great sorrow, the news of my brother-in-law's sudden death (1963, 43).

A more comprehensive example of the Jungian method is Jane Wheelwright's portrayal of the last six months of the life of a terminal cancer patient named Sally (1981). The patient is 37 years old, married, and a mother of two children. She had contracted breast, ovarian, and bone cancer, and her primary treatment consisted of surgery and chemotherapy. Formerly attractive and extroverted, Sally had become emaciated with pain by the time Wheelwright met her.

Sally continually rages against her husband Jim, and she is frequently depressed and self-deprecating. She wants to die but remains ambivalent about it. Sally admits: "Sometimes I dream of a white boat gliding across the water. It's death coming for me. I want to get on that boat and at the same time I don't want to" (22). The ambivalence about her impending death makes her depressed, but she reacts with increased activity. Wheelwright cautions Sally that her activism blocks messages from the unconscious (23).

Early in the therapy Sally has a big dream:

> I came upon a Sumerian Tower with great ramps zig-zagging to the top. It was also Southern California State College overlooking the University of Southern California. I had to climb to the top; it was a horrifying ordeal. When I got there I looked below, and throughout the city I saw buildings from the Sumerian, Romanesque, Gothic, and ancient Indian eras. There was a large, elegant book lying open before me. It was handsomely illustrated with architectural details of these buildings, of their friezes and sculptures. I awakened, terrorized by the height of the tower (28).

In Wheelwright's view, the dream conveys a pent-up need of the unconscious to speak from Sally's center, which touches the streams of humanity. The mountain symbolizes aspiration; the tower is the nucleus of herself; and the city the sphere of herself. The book suggests a need for knowledge. Ascent to the tower equals descent to the unconscious. The terror of the pinnacle of her ascent means that the Self seeks change, but the ego wants to cling.

Shortly thereafter, Sally dreams of

> driving along the edge of the ocean in a station wagon. It was a beautiful scene at dusk. I heard a meow coming from the back seat, and when I turned around I saw a tiny kitten. It looked just like Cyrano, our cat; it was exactly the same type and color. I wondered if I could persuade Jim to let me keep it (36).

Wheelwright interprets this ocean dream as a compensation for the tower dream. Whereas the tower dream expresses Sally's dominating rational personality, the ocean dream brings out the kitten which represents feminine, instinctual nature. Sally learns that whoever is cut off from her instinctual nature becomes vulnerable to disease. The kitten also represents an instinct to flee death.

Throughout this phase of therapy, family tensions persist in Sally's life. She feels alienated from her mother, who drinks heavily and frequently loses consciousness. Since her mother is neither caring nor loving, Sally needs an older, wiser woman, who bears the archetype of the Self. Sally's husband is usually away, which brings anger and resentment. She had not enjoyed sexual intercourse for two and one half years and, as a result, she developed a suicide wish. Sally explains that when she had met her husband, her attraction was mainly sexual. She was raised to believe that sexual desire was against religious faith; so when she married, she lost her faith in God.

During one of Jim's absences, Sally dreams of being on a beach beside a body of water:

> I had to cross this bay on a surf board that was like a raft; I had to paddle it with my hands the way surfers do. It was a huge ordeal, a supreme effort, but somehow I managed to get across. When I arrived on the other shore, I felt relieved and triumphant. Jim met me there and told me he appreciated what I had done, but that for some reason beyond his control I had to go back (93).

Sally awakens before knowing whether or not she had returned from the other shore. At the personal level the dream dramatizes the conflict with her husband; she is sent back because he knows she will die. More profoundly, the dream shows the need to reunite with her husband and to discover her true female selfhood (156).

Midway in the study, Wheelwright points out that the cumulative effect of the dreams is to release pent-up emotion. Sally's masculine-rational need for control creates the pent-up emotion. Unless it is discharged constructively, it will erupt in volcanic explosions. Wheelwright interprets volcanic explosions as collisions of opposites, and so Sally's task is to unify the opposites. In my reading, the opposites are not precisely defined.

At last, Sally enters a hospital, and Jim still has not visited her. Nightly, she screams: "Mother, Mother" (192). She dreams of being persecuted by Nazi terror and of arid soil and barren land. These two images convey victimization and depression, respectively. Sally complains of guilt for getting cancer: "You feel as though you're being punished for some horrendous crime you committed, yet you don't know what the crime was" (200). Consequently, Sally becomes obsessed with evil and at the same time, she seems to exist in a dark tunnel.

Wheelwright says that tunnels appear in dreams of people who feel stuck, who do not know where they are going. She insists that Sally must accept the dark tunnel within her. For this evil is the dark side of God, and the darkness sends cancer and death. Yet Sally cannot accept the darkness within her nor understand how darkness produces light and evil good. In this struggle she fears being unable to breath, which is the same as the fear of death (260).

Sally reports her last dream shortly before her death: "I was a palm tree, the middle one of three trees. An earthquake was about to occur that would destroy all life, and I didn't want to be killed by the quake" (269). Wheelwright associates the palm tree with the Sumerian Tower of Sally's first big dream. She is correct in the sense that Assyrian tablets of 800 B.C.E. identify the palm tree with the tree of life. In the Jungian perspective of this case the tree symbolizes the union of male and female, so that Sally has become the mother "who gives life and lays it to rest" (270). As a palm tree, Sally has returned to the regenerative unconscious, from which she had come.

Wheelwright points out that the earthquake would be the cancer, which Sally fears will destroy her house, i.e. her body. Ironically, Sally died by pneumonia; therefore, she escaped the earthquake she feared so much. However, her unconscious had actually prepared her for death by bringing her close to the earthquake archetype.

Finally, Jane Wheelwright's sensitive account of Sally's death clearly illumines the symbolism of terminal cancer, but I believe the analysis conceals or misses some vital material. By assigning priority to the archetypes, the Jungian analyst is inclined to omit instinctual drive needs and tendencies. To conclude this section I sketch a tentative reinterpretation, based upon the paroxysmal-participatory pattern.

Ascent to the mountain, in the tower dream, expresses Sally's need for ego expansion, for exaltation of her power of being. Through the tower dream Sally strives for participation in social and metaphysical reality. This need belongs to the ego, but it is activated by the cancer as a life-threatening event. The need for expansion is offset by the tendency to cling to the past which also originates in the cancer. The impulse to cling promotes depression and ambivalence.

When Sally dreams of going to the ocean, she reveals a need for healing and restitution. The ocean may be viewed as the collective unconscious, but it does not so much compensate the tower dream, as Wheelwright says, but complements it. Descent is a paroxysmal equivalent of ascent; both symbolize shock events.

Arriving at the distant shore, in the surfboard dream, suggests a momentary state of integration. It is only a potential state, since Sally must return to this shore, to the ordinary world because of her husband's command. He is the condition for her attaining wholeness; and unless the marital conflict is resolved, Sally's striving for participation will be blocked. Healing is not dependent on the interpretation of dreams but on the resolution of unconscious conflict in the marriage.

The crucial insight is that Sally conceals pent-up emotion. The therapeutic task is to release her rage and seek forgiveness. It is not to unite opposites but to make restitution of the marital resentments. To interpret emotional explosions as collisions of opposites, as the Jungian does, is to miss the hidden paroxysmality. Volcanic eruptions symbolize the discharge of crude emotions and a need for restitution. Sally's experience demonstrates that suppressed anger is a symptom of the cancer experience.

The same pent-up emotion lies behind her obsession with evil, a feeling of having committed a crime long ago, and sense of guilt. Reflecting on his epilepsy, Dostoevsky has made the same point in a letter: "I often feel very depressed. It is a sort of abstract depression, as if I had committed a crime against someone" (Frank and Goldstein 1987, 237). Along with the fear of suffocating to death, which also tormented Dostoevsky, all of these factors are psychic equivalents of paroxysmal-epileptiform seizures. Sally's life has built up intense anger, hatred, jealousy, and her cancer signifies punishment for these Cain emotions. Her sad plight is further enhanced by the failure of her parents and husband to support her.

Consequently, the earthquake in the last dream is the eruption of crude Cain affect. Her fear of being killed by the earthquake shows a need for restitution, a need which has not been satisfied. Sally's becoming a palm tree is actually a defense against the volcanic eruption. Although Wheelwright is certainly correct in linking the palm tree with a union of opposites, in ancient Mesopotamia such a union was reserved for the gods and not humans. Since Sally is human and not divine, her palm tree becomes a sign of death, a failure to achieve an exalted power of being. Historically, the palm tree has evolved through Hebrew-Christian civilization as the "dry tree," which is a symbol of death (Peebles 1923, 78). Without resolving her rage and experiencing forgiveness, Sally's drive for participation in social and metaphysical reality turns into a tragedy.

IV. FAMILIAL DEATH VISIONS

Leopold Szondi contributed to modern thought the notion of a distinctly ancestral or familial dream. The breakthrough came in 1916, when Szondi was a 23 year old medical student and serving as a medic in the Austro-Hungarian army. After being wounded in combat, he went to Vienna for convalescence, and there he fell in love with a language teacher, who was a blonde, of Saxon and Aryan descent. He recalls:

> One night I awoke from a dream, in which my parents discussed the sad destiny of my eldest half-brother. He had studied medicine in Vienna more than 30 years before me, and he had also fallen in love with a language teacher, who was even of blonde, Saxon, and Aryan descent. He had to marry her and give up the medical exam. His marriage was not happy (Szondi 1963, 525).

Through this ancestral dream Szondi realized that he was repeating a familial fate pattern. Instead, he wanted to live his own life; so on the next morning he left Vienna and returned to his regiment.

In the course of his later medical practice, Szondi came to understand that images of the ancestors occupy the familial unconscious, and they become manifest in dreams. The ancestral dream corresponds to the genetic fact that the goal of forbearers is to survive in the lives of their descendants (Szondi 1963, 79-81). As a therapist, Szondi was concerned to help the patients work through hereditary disorders that were displayed in dreams, because these had a bearing upon the decision-making of the individual.

Other than Szondi's published work, it is difficult to find documentation of ancestral dreams in modern literature. However, we have cited, in chapter one, Dostoevsky's dream, on July 6, 1864, in which he dreamed of his deceased father, "and his old mother entered, my granny, and all my ancestors." Meanwhile, Hawaiian culture maintains a documented tradition of familial visions. Deceased relatives appear in clear visual and tactual form, usually during a descendant's crisis, and they mandate personal change or proper behavior (MacDonald and Oden 1977).

Otherwise, the most accessible source is the evidence initially compiled in the nineteenth century by the British Society for Psychical Research. Although Frederic Myers began to document familial dreams, another member of the society went on to publish a collection of death-bed visions. William Barrett, Professor of Physics in Dublin, published his material in 1926, and his work was subsequently reissued (1986). Barrett provides a helpful classification of different kinds of visions.

He describes what should be called apparitions of deceased relatives and friends by those who are dying. In some cases the dying had already known of the death, and, in others, they learned of the death while they are dying. Whether their death were known or not, when beholding a deceased relative, one tends to brighten up with joy and ecstasy. The following example has been carefully and critically witnessed by a nurse:

I recall the death of a woman (Mrs. Brown, aged 36) who was the victim of that most dreadful disease, malignant cancer. Her sufferings were excruciating, and she prayed earnestly that death might speedily come to her and end her agony. Suddenly her sufferings appeared to cease; the expression of her face, which a moment before had been distorted by pain, changed to one of radiant joy. Gazing upwards, with a glad light in her eyes, she raised her hands and exclaimed, "Oh, mother dear, you have come to take me home, I am so glad." And in another moment her physical life had ceased (29).

A familial apparition may disclose the fact that a loved one has attained forgiveness in death:

> The dying man…suddenly looked up, opened his eyes wide, and
> looking at the side of the bed opposite to where his wife was,
> exclaimed, "Why, Mother, here is Tom [recently deceased son],
> and he is all right, no marks on him [from a fatal railway
> accident]. Oh, he looks fine." Then after another silence he
> said, "And here's Nance too." A pause, then "Mother, she is
> all right, she has been forgiven" (50).

Barrett explains that the man could die after learning of the forgiveness
of his daughter. She had given birth to a child out of wedlock and died,
after which the baby was born. She had no time to repent.

Barrett records several cases featuring what Frederic Myers called
"travelling clairvoyance," in which the dying behold living persons at a
distance and, occasionally, they share reciprocal visions. For example,
a woman is terminally ill but says she cannot die, until she sees her
children who live in another city. This happens, and then after ten
minutes, she announces: "I am ready now; I have been with my
children" (83). Barrett points out that when notes taken at the place of
death and of the children's residence were compared, the day, hour, and
minute were the same.

Barrett's cases demonstrate an acceleration and expansion of thought
at the brink of death. The mind becomes more alert and aware. Such
enhanced mental activity occurs clearly in the case of Jack, a deaf mute,
who is dying with rheumatic fever. His hands and fingers are so swollen
that he cannot gesture, but, while lying on his back, suddenly

> his face lighted up with the brightest of smiles. After a little
> while Jack awoke and used the words "Heaven" and "beautiful"
> as well as he could by means of his lips and facial expression.
> As he became more conscious he also told us in the same
> manner that his brother Tom and his sister Harriet were coming
> to see him (100).

Since they lived in a distant city, this knowledge had to come from his
clairvoyance. After Jack's partial recovery, "he told us that he had been
allowed to see into Heaven and to hear most beautiful music."

Barrett does not develop a general theory of death-bed visions, but
he points to a "*transcendental self* of the subject,…independent of the

fundamental units of the physical world—matter, time, and space" (169). The transcendental self emerges in the face of death and achieves a psychic relatedness with other selves, whether living or dead, by means of telepathy. Within a transcendental relatedness the space-time, causal world of the living is relativized. Barrett's brief description of the transcendental self is virtually identical to Myers' subliminal self and Jung's Self, and similar to Szondi's pontifical selfhood.

V. "TAKE-AWAY" VISIONS

Barrett's seminal study remained unexamined for about fifty years, until Karlis Osis and Erlendur Haraldsson published an influential study of death-bed visions (1977). On the basis of one thousand terminal patients in the United States and India, they found death-bed visions to be authentic and meaningful factors in dying. One of their major concerns was to distinguish visions from hallucinations. Hallucinations are produced by the sick brain as defenses against stressors. Brain disease, uremic poisoning, 103°F temperature, and drugs are specific causes of hallucinations. Sensory content of hallucinations tends to be this-worldly, unclear, and variable.

In contrast, visions manifest a clear and coherent consciousness, "otherworldly" content obtained by telepathy or clairvoyance, which is consistently uniform. Although visions may mix occasionally with hallucinations, they are fundamentally independent of physiological and pathological processes. While the authors' definitions are conceptually consistent, their argument is flawed by frequently interchanging terms of hallucinations and apparitions.

Nevertheless, they observe that most visions last a short time, whether five, 15, or 30 minutes (61). After the vision ends, the patient dies relatively quickly, usually within an hour or two. The closer to the time of death the vision is, the more likely it will reveal otherworld quality. Primary contents are living persons, the dead, and mythic or religious figures. About half of all visions have a "take-away" function, in which deceased relatives arrive to escort the patient to another world (67).

Normally, dying patients respond positively to the escorts. Their faces brighten up, and they become elated or transfigured. Momentary fear, anxiety, or depression may be felt, but these tend to be transitory. The "take-away" quality is the mandate that causes the mood elevation of the patient. Visions are distributed equally among males and females, young and old, educated and uneducated. Higher education may enhance understanding of the vision, but it is not the cause. Similarly, a prior belief in life after death may be a contributing factor but not the cause of the vision.

Osis and Haraldsson contend that the terminal patient's positive affects come from a clear, coherent grasp of a real other world (80). Otherworldly states have an intentionality irreducible to patients' needs and desires. The authors also concede that the mind loosens or dissociates from the body in the face of death (128, 131). They draw an analogy of dissociation from schizophrenia, but in light of Frederic Myers' work and Dostoevsky's experience a better analogy for mental dissociation at death would be epilepsy, in which ecstatic joy is experienced. Nevertheless, the argument of Osis and Haraldsson clearly deviates from that of psychoanalysis, according to which elation comes from regression to the pleasure principle, from a temporary suspension of the reality principle, and from a return to infantile omnipotence. In contrast, Osis and Haraldsson maintain that the joy of the "take-away" visions derives from an otherworld beyond the reality principle.

VI. ASSESSMENT OF VISIONS

In current discussions, Robert Kastenbaum offers a critique of death-bed visions in his text-book (1991, 324-325). He charges that the research mode of the Osis and Haraldsson study is impaired by its retrospective approach. Data were actually recollections gathered by health care-givers, who lacked training in research methods. Some of their recollections went back many years and might have become vague or unreliable. Some of the witnesses even disagreed with one another and, therefore, were too subjective.

Kastenbaum emphasizes the personal needs of the patient. Since dying patients tend to deny their own deaths, it is difficult for them to attain acceptance. As biological creatures concerned with survival, humans cope with death by needs and projections. On the one hand, we deny death; and, on the other, we project the survival of death in the form of a desired immortality. Impending death creates a splitting within the patient. Part of the self denies death, while another part of the self communicates a fantasy of survival by means of desire. Hence, desire for immortality arises from the pleasure principle with its defense against a real threat of death. Kastenbaum's argument presupposes Freud's opinion that the unconscious knows no death and his conception of the brain as a closed physical system.

Kastenbaum's argument also exemplifies the "split-off" phase, a stage of terminal illness recognized by psychoanalysis. Esther Dreifuss-Kattan defines the "split-off" phase:

> Two opposite ideas are verbalized: one, a full realization of the closeness of death; the other, a faith in surviving, often expressed in vivid fantasies about the future. The perception of this split and the psychological handling of it is, for those surrounding the patient, extremely difficult, since the split stands in opposition to the reality principle that governs our ordinary, day-to-day existence,...(1990, 102).

Dreifuss-Kattan contends that the suspension of the reality principle activates the timeless mother-child union and its rich fantasy sources. The "split-off" phase is irrational but not psychotic, because the dying patient acquires a heightened awareness, while ego functions remain intact. Evidence of the nonpsychotic character of the "splitting" appears in writings or drawings produced by terminal cancer patients. Such works embody creative fantasies that offer hope as forms of reparation. Creativity nullifies the negative effects of disease, such as pain, and draws out symbolic images from the unconscious. Symbolism makes restitution and strives for healing in the dying process.

The combined arguments of Kastenbaum and Dreifuss-Kattan are compelling and clinically sound. Certainly, the "split-off" phase comes amid the stage of visionary activity in terminal illness. However, the "split-off" phase has been interpreted differently by Jungian psychology. It is acknowledged when a patient becomes withdrawn and demoralized, or seems far-away and detached, as though no human relationship had any more meaning. The "split-off" phase means the cessation of the wishing and fearing ego as well as the breakthrough of a spiritual consciousness (von Franz 1987, 111, 116-117). The spiritual consciousness represents the Self, which transcends time, space, causality, and survives bodily death. Reparative processes of terminal illness are also breakthroughs of the timeless realm of the psyche. The Jungian interpretation has the virtue of recognizing a positive transcendental function rather than a regression.

Having reviewed the clinical context of death-bed visions, it is necessary to discuss an evaluation. First, the Osis and Haraldsson study is, admittedly, retrospective and subjective, as Kastenbaum insists. However, when reading the vision literature as a whole, this objection cannot be maintained; for data on death-bed visions have been carefully collected and rigorously analyzed, particularly by the British scholars in the nineteenth century. Methodologies employed by Myers, Barrett and their colleagues came from the so-called "hard" sciences. Eye-witness accounts were verified, making the body of literature as a whole reliable. Ironically, Kastenbaum confesses that he has witnessed several death-bed visions, and he continues to wonder (1991, 325). His admission implies that death-bed visions are dramatic, overpowering, and not easily forgotten. To ensure accuracy witnesses should simply record or write out what is occurring.

Second, the purported need to deny death for the sake of survival may be challenged in light of evolutionary genotropism. As defined in chapter two, genotropism is a reciprocal attraction between carriers of the same or related genes. This means that relatives share higher concentrations of identical or related genes compared to general populations. The reason for such genetic clustering is that genes promote their own survival by creating reciprocal attraction between carriers. Organisms have the tendency to select similar or identical genetic types, whether genealogically related or not. Gene relatedness is a fundamental fact of evolving nature, and it precedes phenotypic traits of appearance, race, and class.

Genotropism illumines a basic fact that serves as a cornerstone of the theory of natural selection, namely, the experience of altruism. Within the animal kingdom animals allow themselves to die on behalf of a relative or offspring, and they expose themselves to mortal danger in defense against territorial intruders (Smith 1964). For example, a parent animal may give up food for an offspring, when resources are scarce. Birds engage in apparent "suicide" attack behavior toward a territorial intruder, who threatens the family nest during the breeding season. While the parent animal might die, at least half of the genes survive in the descendant's gene pool. For the same reason, when a human dies in order to save family members, copies of one's own or related genes will survive (Dawkins 1976, 97).

A corresponding willingness to die among humans occurs in the clinical pattern called "predilection to death," involving persons who know they are dying and may even predict the time of death accurately. They look forward to a reunion of familial relationships in death and, consequently, feel neither grief nor fear (Weisman and Hackett 1961). Predilection cases should not be confused with "Voodoo" death or with suicide, which involve lethality and tools. Predilection to death is a natural willingness to die, motivated by the needs to escape unmanageable pain and to resume a love relationship in death.

Within the history of religions the predilection to die correlates with the "dying at will," as practiced in Hawaii and other Pacific cultures (Sato 1964, Cooke 1976). One dies intentionally and naturally, without starvation, tools, or disease. Dying at will is done mainly by older Hawaiians, who maintain the beliefs of the traditional ancestral religion and who claim that non-Hawaiians are unable to perform it. One version of the "dying at will" is the Hawaiian "take my life instead" ritual. When one is seriously ill, another member of the family prays to die instead and does die. Normally, it is a child who suffers a life-threatening illness, and an older relative dies in his or her place. One Hawaiian scholar relates that "her nephew was awfully sick, and my great-grandmother chose to die that he might live. He lived. She died" (Pukui 1972, 134).

Dying often coincides with a vision of an ancestor, most frequently a grandparent or grandchild. Records of visions are kept at Queen Liliuokalani Children's Center in Honolulu, and one typical example follows: "TuTu sat up in bed and said, 'Look! the relatives [Aumakua] are waiting for me!' and then she was gone" (ibid, 13).

In traditional Hawaiian religion the ancestors belong to four broad groups of descent, each one correlated with a primal element: Pele, goddess of the volcano (fire); thunder and lightning (air); sharks (water); and turtles and lizards (earth). When received by the ancestors, the dying patient is transfigured in an appropriate manner (Kamakau 1964, 64-65). For example, descendants of Pele envision columns of fire. These lines of familial descent are designated by paroxysmal symbols, implying that familial relatedness copes with the shock suffering of death.

Altogether, the combined evidence of dying at will, predilection to death, and biological altruism suggests that genotropism operates in death. The natural willingness to die is motivated by an unconscious, genotropic attraction to close family members.

Third, it is surely correct to emphasize as Kastenbaum does, that dying patients face death in terms of a need. Psychoanalysis assigns biological priority to the sexual drive, and since it ceases at death, then death must be denied. My question is: What need takes priority in terminal illness? As stated above, preservation of the individual organism is not absolute in evolution, since in times of mortal danger altruism compels a willingness to die. This fact conforms to the paroxysmal pattern rather than the sexual drive. Terminal illness activates the paroxysmal pattern in defense against the onset of death. This defense takes shape through dreams and visions, through the symbolism of air, earth, fire, and water, and through the acceleration of the psyche. Following the psychiatric study of epilepsy, paroxysmality must be distinguished from sexuality.

The root need of the paroxysmal pattern is that of atonement. The intent of accelerating thought at the brink of death is to make restitution as a condition of wholeness. Once the restitution need is satisfied, one opens up to a transcendent dimension and seeks to strip away the body. Going beyond the body fulfills the primal drive for metaphysical participation in fundamental reality. This paroxysmal-participatory mode usually rotates into the dying person's foreground as a "split-off" phase.

Traditional Hawaiian religion provides a clear illustration of the paroxysmal-participatory phase of dying. One turns toward the ancestors who dwell in the eternal.

There is a sea of time, so vast man cannot know its boundaries, so fathomless man cannot plumb its depths. Into this dark sea plunge the spirits of men, released from their earthly bodies. The sea becomes one with the sky and the land and the fiery surgings that rise from deep in the restless earth. For this is the measureless expanse of all space. This is the timelessness of all time. This is eternity (Pukui 1972, 35).

The island represents the waking ego, the ancestors the familial unconscious, and the ocean the collective unconsciousness. Freely joining the ancestors transfigures the dead and relativizes the oceanic horizon into the eternal.

CHAPTER FIVE:
DREAMS AND VISIONS OF GRIEF

I. IMAGERY AND GRIEF WORK

Frederic Myers observed that dreams and visions appear to bereaved survivors for one year after a death, and he justified this observation by grounding dreams and visions in the veridical afterimage. Myers' contention accords well with mourning even though he did not conceptualize the grieving process as such. When grief became understood clinically in the twentieth century, dreams and visions were relatively neglected. The principal theoretical reason was in "Mourning and Melancholia" (1917) Sigmund Freud formulated grief primarily as a process of separation from the deceased (1959 C.P.IV). Attention to dreams and visions might inhibit the necessary process of detachment; for according to psychoanalysis they exhibit a failure of reality testing and infantile regression. In psychoanalysis the imagery of dreams and visions is a hallucinatory retention of the lost object.

Essentially, grief is a personal response to the loss of a dependent or interdependent relationship. Despite Freud's pioneering insight, the principal theorist of grief in the twentieth century is Erich Lindemann, whose classic study of survivors of the Cocoanut Grove fire in Boston established the definitions of acute normal, delayed, and abnormal grief (1944). Basic to acute grief is a common syndrome, comprising bodily distress, specifically, "waves lasting from 20 minutes to an hour at a time," along with tightness in the throat, choking, difficulties in breathing, need for sighing, feeling of emptiness, powerlessness, and mental tension or pain (141-142). These bodily symptoms co-exist with guilt, hostility, loss of behavioral patterns, identification with traits of the deceased, and preoccupation with a mental image of the deceased.

Lindemann points out that a morbid reaction could take place, if the mental image were to replace grieving by the deceased, whose senses would be altered by the shock of death. "There is commonly a slight sense of unreality, a feeling of increased emotional distance from other people (sometimes they appear shadowy or small), and there is intense preoccupation with the image of the deceased" (142). The latter is "a vivid visual image of his presence," in the words of one widow (143). At the same time, the bereaved displays increased activity, mobility, and speech; but these are not necessarily well-organized or goal-directed. These characteristics are expected to appear during the first seven or ten days after the death, which is the period of the most intense grief.

After this initial intensity of grief diminishes somewhat, the bereaved faces a series of tasks, known as grief work. Generalizing on Lindemann's papers, grief work consists of (1) real acceptance of the actual fact of death; (2) feeling the pain; (3) balanced recollection of the life and death of the deceased; (4) gradual separation of the bereaved from the deceased; and (5) resumption of interpersonal and social activity, even while acknowledging the finality of the loss (1944, 1976, 1980).

Central to grief work is the change of the meaning of the deceased, specifically, the transition from a physical being to a spiritual presence within the bereaved. This shift is both difficult and constructive, because the loss hurts and sometimes requires taking on a new familial or social role. Although the person has departed, he or she remains in the minds and hearts of the survivors. Lindemann calls this change resurrection, and he defines it as a "fervent effort to resurrect or make permanent what the deceased person had to offer...." (1976, 202) Resurrection includes a reallocation of the functions of the deceased in the network of survivors, internalization of one or more of these functions, and actualizing these for oneself. Avoidance of the vivid imagery, accompanying these tasks, obstructs resurrection and delays or disturbs the grief work.

Even though Lindemann recognized the significant role of imagery in grief work, only a few clinicians have examined it since his death in 1972. One reason for the relative neglect is a confusion in definitions. For example, in a study of 227 Welsh widows and 66 widowers Dewi Rees explains that "a sense of the presence" of the deceased spouse was reported in 46.7% of deaths. He writes that the "term 'hallucination' is used to include 'a sense of the presence of the dead person,' in addition to visual, auditory, and tactile hallucinations" (Rees 1975, 66). His definition is tautological, because it confuses the meanings of presence and hallucinations.

Despite the logical and semantic confusion, the Rees study contains significant empirical data. Along with "the sense of presence," 14% had visual "hallucinations," 13.3% auditory, and 2.7% tactile. "Hallucinations" were more common for those who had happy marriages, with children, and who belonged to professional and managerial classes. Rees judged the "hallucinations" to be normal and common, unassociated with illness or abnormality, but helpful in the grieving process. To illustrate, some of his case material is quoted below:

"He seems so close" (widowed 7 years). "I heard, how shall I put it, sounds of consolation for the first three months" (widowed 26 years). "I feel him guiding me" (widowed 15 years).

"I fancy, if I left here, I would be running away from him. Lots of people wanted me to go, but I just couldn't. I often hear him walking about. He speaks quite plainly. He looks younger, just as he was when he was all right, never as he was ill" (widowed 9 months). (69)

If these presences were helpful to the bereaved, then they should not be described as hallucinations. As defined in chapter four, hallucinations leave people unchanged. Since these phenomena facilitate grief work, they should be given a positive reference that respects the intent of dreams and visions. Presence is an appropriate term, and it has been defined as an "experience in which the subject, in clear consciousness, suddenly becomes aware of the presence of another person in the immediate vicinity, although the subject may in reality be alone, or in the company of others" (Thompson 1980, 628). Despite the tautology in the definition, the author attempts an original formulation by using the German term *Anwesenheit* for "presence." He distinguishes it from sensory objects, hallucinations, and delusions. Usually, the identity of the presence is that of a deceased relative, who offers comfort but sometimes a threat. Presence comes involuntarily, in the manner of an epileptic aura, and it is normal in grief. Therefore, the presence, if properly defined, facilitates the resurrection phase of grief work.

From the perspective of ego psychology, presence conforms to the dynamics of introjective-participation. After the death, the bereaved person incorporates the image of the "deceased" through identification. Death releases an unconscious introjection mechanism that works like a camera, photographing images of the lost object (Szondi 1956, 199). The affective and traumatic impact of the loss influences the sharpness and clarity of the photographic image (*Hyper-Introjektion*). The bereaved maintain the images in a mental album. The primary intent of the introjection is to restore the relationship, because ego states obey the primal drive for participation in social and metaphysical reality. As will be discussed below, dreams and visions of grief may also introject the presence of a deceased ancestor. A familial introjection bears upon the role of decision-making in grief work, such as ending mourning or making vocational choices.

Whether personal or familial, introjective-participation means that fundamentally grief work is a matter of relatedness. Even though a physical being has died, the relationship has not. The relationship continues after death, and grief work means that it must change. Completed grief work signifies the achievement of a spiritual relatedness with the deceased, or resurrection, as Lindemann would say, as well as an adaptation to social and metaphysical reality. Complicated or incomplete grief work indicates a maladaptive response to reality, fixation on the introjected object, and disorganized behavior. Complicated grief work remains a distinct possibility, because the loss of a dependency relationship, even if liberating, carries a hidden depressive mood (Szondi 1972, 194).

Similarly, Jungian psychology recognizes that mourning is partly detachment from the lost object but mainly the creation of a new relationship with the dead. The medium of bereavement relatedness is the creative imagination. Drawing upon the work of Jung and Corbin, Greg Mogenson has developed an imaginal view of mourning as "greeting the angels" (1992). He means that after the separation phase of grief work the dead reproduce themselves as essential, imaginal beings, who are autonomous and who should be respected as ends in themselves. The imaginal forms need not be interpreted but simply incorporated into the living. As long as the dead are internalized by the bereaved, then the latter will not be projecting or introjecting the lost object in the mode of abnormal grief. Rather mourning is soul-making; for the dead dwell in the soul like photographs in a family album (24). Grief develops the images in the film of death.

Although Szondi had already stressed the notions of the photograph album and ancestral presence, the Jungian approach is a constructive affirmation of the adaptive aspect of grief work. However, the Jungian method tends to neglect the critical psychodynamic phase of grief work, such as ambivalence and despair. What if the deceased were greeted not as an angel but as a terror of the night? What if the dead were felt as hauntings? In such cases, the analysis should examine the quality of the relationship between the bereaved and the deceased.

Mogenson has written an original and stimulating study of grief, stressing the transition from relatedness to imaginal being. However, his selection of case material omits, in some areas, specifically death-related imagery. For example, in his chapter on bereavement dreams, the examples chosen derive from a divorce rather than from death (89-97). Divorce yields a being who has departed but not one who has died.

In conclusion, hallucinations, presences, dreams, visions, and apparitions emerge in the grieving process, and all but hallucinations contribute to the completion of grief work. It is imperative to discover and interpret these imaginal phenomena, because in contemporary society often the bereaved receive no guidance from established social or religious rituals. The demonstrated value of traditional mourning rituals is that they channel feelings aroused by the death, prescribe constructive behavior, and help the bereaved to reintegrate with familial or social groups. As substitutes for rituals, dreams and visions appear and provide a subjective narrative framework. In whatever form they take, bereavement images reflect the nature of the relationships involved. They obey the law of participation.

II. BEREAVEMENT DREAMS

Sigmund Freud interpreted bereavement dreams as fulfillments of a death wish (1953, S.E.IV, 249). The death wish is not satisfied in the present time but in the past. Hence, to dream that one's mother has died, after her actual death, satisfies an earlier death wish against her. While this type of situation may occur, this theory cannot apply to all cases but only to those in which the grief entails an intense sense of guilt.

In contrast, Jung viewed bereavement dreams in terms of the process of self-realization. The dream displays the deceased in his or her primal form, objectively, and devoid of projections and emotions. Jung achieved this insight, after the death of his wife Emma, who appeared in a dream, having the quality of a vision:

> She stood at some distance from me, looking at me squarely. She was in her prime, perhaps about thirty, and wearing the dress which had been made for her many years before by my cousin the medium. It was perhaps the most beautiful thing she had ever worn. Her expression was neither joyful nor sad, but, rather, objectively wise and understanding, without the slightest emotional reaction....(1961, 296)

Jung's experience offers an excellent example of a bereavement dream as a constructive event, but we do not know whether the dream says something about the nature of his marriage or about the grief process in general. To supplement Jung's basic insight a theory of bereavement dreams should acknowledge the respective personal, familial, and collective/archetypal regions of the unconscious, and indicate how these bear upon grief work.

Bereavement dreams can arrive shortly before a death or sometimes after, possibly a few days after or several weeks. Dreams signify the fact that, although someone has died, the relationship with the bereaved continues. Dreams reflect the fundamental relational constitution of human beings. Generally, the content of a normal bereavement dream is clear, undistorted, and the deceased is portrayed in a youthful, healthy, or nonterminal manner (Gorer 1973, 430). Should the deceased be presented as sick, aged, or dying, along with unclear, distorted lines, then the dream reflects an on-going complication in the relationship with the deceased. Such a dream signifies that grief work is either inhibited or incompleted. When the deceased has no shape at all, then the bereaved has not brought the relationship into self-consciousness. A severe conflict may be present unconsciously, and participation is blocked in some way.

In the remainder of this section some examples of bereavement dreams are presented and discussed. The first comes from a former student of mine who had a dream, recurring three times during her father's death. Three days before his death, she had the dream twice, once in the morning and once in the evening. The dream appeared once after his death. On each occasion the dream was the same. The significance of a thrice-repeated dream is that conflict is being resolved and brought up to the threshold of consciousness (Benz 1968, 15). As an illustration, Dostoevsky's dream of his father, his ancestors, and the father's diagnosis of his tuberculosis also came three times (Frank and Goldstein 1987, 353-354).

The student describes her dream as follows:

It was late at night and my whole family was together in our living room. I was standing in the dining room watching my family. My father was sitting on the sofa and my two sisters were on either side of him. My mother was sitting on a chair next to them. My father was playing with my dog who was very old and feeble. It had been a long time since my dog was well enough to play ball, and he was running around like a puppy again. We were all laughing at him as he tried to get the ball away from my father. My father acted as he had when he was well, smiling and happy. I could see his face very clearly and I felt good seeing him looking so well.

I was standing away from my family looking and talking to them. I can't remember what I was saying, but I believe I was complaining about something being wrong. My father looked up at me and said: "M., don't worry. Everything's going to be all right. Don't worry." I remember feeling greatly relieved....

The dreamer's waking consciousness recedes, while familial figures take center stage. The father's change from a dying to a healthy state in the dream signifies surpassing the threshold. His message of consolation, presented as a mandate, indicates positive adaptation in the dreamer's grieving. The key archetypal symbol is the dog. In reality the dog was old and feeble, but in the dream the dog becomes a puppy again.

The appearance of the dog is an archetypal affirmation of normal grief work. In Old Iranian religion and Zoroastrianism the dog is the mediator between the living and the dead (Boyce 1989, 144). Zoroastrian Creation Theology ranks dogs next to humans in order of value. In the Hindu Vedas two dogs are messengers of Yama, god of the dead; and they find those who are about to die and take them to the other life. In Zoroastrianism two dogs await the soul of the deceased at the Chinvat Bridge. For the dying, the last rites are performed three times. Thus, the three fold appearance of the dream, the ritual use of number three, and the dog reflect the religious culture that developed the symbolism of the bridge.

A second example comes from a former student, whose father died in the fall of 1989. Having been a severe alcoholic, he generated a deep ambivalence in his daughter. She loved him but hated his drinking. In February, 1990, on the night of his birthday, she dreamed that "my father was at my house and he was a recovered alcoholic. He said he was going to be fine and he would never leave me again."

Another dream appeared, in which she could not see her father's face clearly but knew it was he:

> He was very ill and had come to apologize to me for never really sharing my childhood and watching me grow through my teen years. He said that it was probably for the best that he wasn't around, because he wouldn't have been much of [a] parent because he was too involved with his drinking.

The house in the first dream represents the dreamer's own psyche, as inferred from Jung's house dream (1961, 158). Both dreams deal with the dreamer's need for attachment to the father. In the first dream the need is satisfied; but in the second it is not, because the absence of the father's face means that the relationship has not achieved self-consciousness. Here the grief is intense, and the sorrow over the father's remorse suggests loneliness, broken bonding, and incomplete grief work. Viewed together, both dreams convey a profound ambivalence.

A third example consists of a series of bereavement dreams reported by the Jungian scholar Marie-Louise von Franz (1987, 111-112, 133, 148). Her father had died suddenly, when she was away from home, and she had the following dream about three weeks after his death:

> It was about ten o'clock in the evening, dark outside. I heard the doorbell ring and "knew" at once somehow that this was my father coming. I opened the door and there he stood with a suitcase.... "I know that I am dead, but may I not visit you?"

I said: "Of course, come in," and then asked, "How are you now?"

Her father explains that he has returned to Vienna, his home-town, that he is studying music and is happy. He says he is only a guest now:

"It is not good for either the dead or the living to be together too long. Leave me now. Good night." And with a gesture he signalled me not to embrace him, but to go. I went into my own room, thinking that I had forgotten to put out the electric stove and that there was a danger of fire. At that moment I woke up, feeling terribly hot and sweating.

Following Jung, she interprets the dream as a statement of the bereavement situation. Her father had died and had become content. The motif of the stove and fire at the end is a compensation for the fact that the dead are cold; i.e. the dead are "split-off" from the living and their warmth and relatedness.

In my view, the meaning of the stove is entirely different, and it bears upon the nature of epilepsy; namely, fire as a psychic equivalent of a latent epileptiform condition (Szondi 1956, 99). The "danger of fire" is the threat of pent-up emotion, triggered by the absence of the father, and probably an upsurge of anger. Waking up hot and sweating designates a post-paroxysmal consequence of an emotional discharge.

Furthermore, about six weeks after his death, she dreamed of her father as healthy and alive, even though she knew he was dead:

He said to me in cheerful excitement, "the resurrection of the flesh is a reality. Come with me, I can show it to you." He started walking toward the cemetery where he was buried. I dreaded to follow him but I did. In the cemetery he walked around and between the graves, observing every one. Suddenly he pointed to a grave and called out. "Here, for instance, come and look." I saw that the earth there had begun to move and I stared in that direction, full of dread that a half-decomposed corpse was about to appear. Then I saw that a crucifix was drilling its way upwards out of the earth. It was about one meter long, golden-green and shining. My father called out, "Look here! *This* is the resurrection of the flesh."

As a Jungian, her starting point is ancient alchemy and the archaic pre-Christian psyche. Accordingly, the green-gold crucifix is animated metal, and in alchemy this symbolizes a union of opposites. The suffering implied in the archetype of the crucifix is that of unreconciled opposites. Hence, the dream portrays the resurrection body as a union of opposites, which is the fulfillment of the self and which is joined to the ego, namely, her father's identity.

I read this dream instead as an expression of grief work. Here resurrection simply means newly completed grief work, as Lindemann has explained, but the crucifix and the dread indicate that the dreamer has not yet made the decisive sacrifice, or break from the deceased, and resumed social interaction. Her grief work is not finished.

Finally, she describes a dream coming five years after her father's death, in which she and her sister jump onto tram number eight, heading for the center of Zürich. They realized that they have made a mistake and are going in the opposite direction. The conductor (*controlleur*) walks through the tram, wearing a hat with the letters EWZ, which designate the Electricity Works of Zürich.

> At the next tram stop we got off and there a taxi drove up near us and out of it—came my father! I knew it was his ghost. When I started to greet him he made a sign not to come too near him and then walked away to the house where he had lived. I called after him. "We don't live there any more." But he shook his head and murmured, "That doesn't matter to me now."

The key dream motifs are the number eight and the conductor (*controlleur*). In alchemy eight is the number of completion, and the "*controlleur*" is associated with the control in spiritualistic seances who mediates between the medium and deceased spirits. Since the "*controlleur*" is from the electrical works, he signifies a transformed frequency of currents. Thus, death as the goal of self-realization is also an energy transformation beyond a certain threshold.

Her insight into the threshold function of the dream contributes to a unified theory of dreamwork, as developed in chapter four, section two. Here I would observe that the three bereavement dreams have had the threshold function of working the grief to that of separation from the deceased. The notion of electrical works relates to that of heat and fire in the first dream, where it means pent-up emotion, such as anger. In this, the third dream, the electricity denotes the sublimation of anger. The dreamer has essentially come to terms with her father's death and is able to live with the anger of his abrupt departure.

Sublimation of anger points to the possibility of restitution, as expressed archetypally. Historically, alchemy did not evolve in complete separation from Christianity; for example, the Lutheran mystic Jacob Boehme used alchemy to interpret the world as alive (Koyré 1968, 45). Thus, the number eight could also refer to the eighth day of Creation or the resurrection. Making a Christian application of the number eight allows the second dream, with the resurrection of the flesh, to cohere with the third dream. Since restitution is a liberating experience, making possible participation in fundamental reality, then the *controlleur* would be the pontifical self which is the inner controller.

III. BEREAVEMENT VISIONS

In the grieving process the sense of presence often comes in the form of a vision. The visionary presence is involuntary, frequently overpowering, and usually consoling; it is neither a sensory object nor a feeling. Since the vision comforts the bereaved, it may appear toward the end of mourning, signifying the completion of grief work. In the following two examples the recipients of the vision do not startle, but in the absence of anxiety achieve a deeper and wider participation.

The first case illustrates how the presence, which comes during a marital crisis, helps a man accept his grandfather's death:

> Suddenly I felt someone behind me, and turned around and, God, it was my grandfather. He was sitting there, perfectly real, and kind of smiled at me. My body felt relaxed, I wasn't shaking any more, and seeing him there was so strange that I wasn't even startled. We just looked at each other, maybe for half a minute, and then he just was gone. I cried for some time, but I felt after that I had made my peace with him. I still missed him, but things were somehow different. *I wasn't carrying him around inside of me*, he was finally gone (Hoyt 1980-1981, 106).

The second example comes from a former student, whose father died on January 26, 1979, when she was nine years old and the youngest child in the family. He died unexpectedly in an automobile accident one wintry night, while returning home from a business trip. The death was so devastating that, for many years, she felt intense anger at the loss and extreme yearning for him. Writing in a paper for me, she explains:

> One night about a year after his death, I was sleeping and was awakened by a voice. I sat up in my bed and my father stood before me. He looked so peaceful and kind, I was not scared or startled, I felt a feeling of security and happiness. He looked at me and said, "I love you, I miss you, and I want you to know that I'm watching over you. If you ever need me I will always be here for you." I blinked my eyes and he was gone.

The next example comes from an interview that I conducted with a terminally ill man on August 27, 1975. After 14 years of marriage, his wife had died on September 4, 1959. About one month later, he received without surprise a vision of his deceased wife, early in the morning while lying in bed awake. He had not been dreaming. He gave me a typed copy of the vision:

> The appearance was of her face and head only. She was looking at me from a few inches from my eyes. The appearance was in a perfect circle filling my whole vision. The shorter hair around her ears and neck appeared to be standing straight out.
> She was smiling slightly. She came to me (or was allowed to breakthrough to me by God) to tell me things, I knew that. The lines in her face probably helped her expressive eyes and smile in making it possible for me to understand so completely her message. Her message was that she was so completely well pleased with me. This was the *overwhelming* feeling that I had. She seemed to say with the most wonderful expression in her eyes. "Everything is all right now."

He began to meditate on this vision for consolation and for hope of reunion in his own death. On March 14, 1961, at 4:00 a.m. he was awakened by the voice of his wife calling to him. "There was no dream with it, just the voice calling clearly as though she might be calling me from the kitchen for me to come to sit down with her for supper."

The cumulative effect of the twice-repeated presence, one visual and the other auditory, was the restoration of his religious faith, as transmitted by his ancestors. He identified with a specific ancestor, a Scottish Presbyterian, who sailed to New Jersey in 1685 in search of religious freedom. Recovery of his ancestral faith helped him to endure the loneliness of dying. The appearance of the wife in a "perfect circle," in the first vision, is a Jungian mandala, suggesting her completed self-realization in death. She had attained her primal form, and his ancestral faith enabled him to participate in her wholeness.

Finally, a series of familial visions, received by a nine year old girl, has been reported by her step-father, one of my former students. A. was nine in the spring of 1992, when her maternal grandmother died. One week after the death, A. was awakened from sleep by a vision of the grandmother. "A. describes her grandmother as she remembers her, in good health, with brown hair and wearing a white dress. A. states her grandmother spoke to her saying that she missed them all and asked A. to say hello to her mother and her brother."

On the next night A. was again awakened from sleep, this time by a deceased paternal grandfather, whom she had never seen:

A. describes her grandfather's appearance with an astonishing resemblance of his actual appearance. A. states that her grandfather was tall, with short brown hair much like her father's, and was wearing a pair of pants with suspenders. A. continues saying that her grandfather was alone and told her "tell your father I miss him."

Two or three weeks later A. was awakened still again by her great grandmother, calling her name and accompanied by an angel. A. sees the grandmother, as she remembers her, healthy and wearing a white dress.

A. describes the angel as being young in her twenties, extremely beautiful with long red hair and green eyes, wearing a white dress with wings protruding from her back. A. said the angel spoke, "Whenever you have fears, don't worry I'll be there." A. tells me that she had a fourth and final visitation one month after her third experience, this time she was awakened from her sleep by the sole presence of the same angel who came before. A. says the angel appeared and asked her how she was doing, and then she left.

My student informs me that the story has an epilogue. A. had attended the funeral of her great grandmother and took home a rose from a bouquet.

> A. placed the rose in a vase filled with water and placed the vase on her bedroom window sill. Naturally, the rose had died within a few days, and the petals had withered away. Over the next few weeks, and parallel to A.'s visitations, the rose stem sprung to life, and to this day it still remains alive.

The rose remained alive, at least, until July, 1992, when I officiated at the wedding of the student and A.'s mother. In my view the angel is an exact projection of the physical features of the mother, and the angel's white dress is the mother's wedding gown. The projected presence of the mother assures the child in facing the momentous change brought about by the wedding. The mother had been divorced for several years and was preparing to be remarried.

The springing to life of the rose is an example of psychokinesis, which psychoanalysis explains as an externalization of aggressive energy, usually by adolescents feeling sexual conflict. The discharge of energy is destructive of objects in the environment. However, the psychoanalytic explanation fails to fit in this case for two reasons: the subject is pre-pubescent and the energy is constructive not destructive.

Meanwhile, the other episodes are genuine ancestral visions, and, in the absence of a convincing psychoanalytic explanation, may have discharged energy that effected the rose. It is already known that dying organisms emit intense electromagnetic energy (Morse with Perry 1992, 142). While this might be too speculative, the projected image of the mother, the ancestral visions, and the new life of the rose express, respectively, the personal, familial, and archetypal unconscious regions of the girl.

IV. TERRORS OF THE NIGHT

When Frederic Myers conceptualized the subliminal self, he acknowledged a phenomenon of nocturnal paralysis, believing it to be a nightmare associated with hysteria (I 1903/1954, 124). It occurred on the border between sleeping and waking, and it produced imagery with so much visual power that it lingered as an afterimage.

A similar observation appears in the new scientific school of dreams. Dream-like forms, called hypnopompic hallucinations, come on arousal from sleep and extend into waking consciousness; and when they combine with sleep paralysis, dread results (Hobson 1988, 8). The neurological reason is that the brain cannot switch instantly from one state to another.

The neurological explanation neglects the personal significance of the phenomena. Clinically, this factor has been identified as a night terror, and, in contrast to the nightmare, it comprises four primary characteristics: (1) feeling of fear or agonizing dread by seeing or hearing an intrusive presence; (2) awakening from sleep; (3) feeling of pressure on the chest to the point of suffocation or strangulation; and (4) becoming paralyzed and unable to move (Hufford 1982, 10-11). The intrusive force may have location, motion, or gender. With the assault by this presence one's eyes open widely, the heart pounds, and one perspires. Nearly all of the victims (90%) are lying on their backs.

Since victims are lying on their backs, psychoanalysis interprets night terrors as projections of repressed sexual or incestuous desires. However, the primary characteristics are epileptiform and, therefore, suggest that the night terrors represent the paroxysmal pattern. In any case, they are neither abnormal nor depressive in themselves, but in the grieving process they pose potential complications for grief work.

To illustrate I select the experience of a former student, a middle-aged woman, who studied with me in the fall semester, 1975. She had married a veteran of the Second World War. Once, in combat, he was hit in the chest by a projectile, and shrapnel remained above the heart. A military physician recommended surgical removal of the shrapnel, when he returned home. He promised he would, but after the war ended, he failed to do so.

In February, 1953 he died of a coronary occlusion. His young widow found herself alone, having to raise their little boy, and manage the household. In a paper for me she wrote: "I functioned in a state of shock. It all seemed unreal. I experienced nausea, loss of appetite, tightness in the throat and chest, and an emptiness as though part of me had died."

For a while, she considered suicide but gave it up with the realization that her son needed at least one parent. She had difficulty making decisions and fervently prayed and wished that her husband might return to help her.

It happened for the first time about two months after his death. A white, ghost-like form appeared to be standing at the foot of my bed. I could feel a presence and I tried desperately to see his face but there was none. It seemed as though he wanted to say something but was unable to and just stood there. The tension of waiting for something to happen frightened me and I found myself trying to scream. The emotion was so real that I didn't realize that I was asleep until my scream awakened me and I found myself sitting straight-up in bed. I could see the vision so clearly that it was difficult for me to believe that my eyes were not opened until I awakened.

Between 1953 and 1975, the presence came regularly. She looked forward to it and tried not to be afraid, but every night she screamed in terror and became paralyzed. Remarkably, this presence, which originally stood at the foot of the bed, began to move slowly toward the corner, turn, and go along the side. Over the span of 22 years, the presence slowly inched toward her. It seemed

to be getting closer and closer and I am afraid to come in contact with it because I fear it will smother me. Recently I have gotten awake with my mouth filled with saliva about to choke on it. If he is coming to take me with him I am only too glad to go. I have been ready for death since his death occurred.

During the same 22 years, but not lasting as long, she had a bereavement dream co-existing with the night terror:

I can see him as clear as can be in his original form but he has never communicated with me. There is always a group of people around and I try to get his attention, but he ignores me. My feelings are hurt and I stand around waiting for him to recognize me and to come toward me but he never does. When I awake I am emotionally distressed.

About two years after the death, she married and eventually bore two more children. The family moved from one city to another within Pennsylvania. Nevertheless, the presence "followed" and visited her at night, always in the same manner. Despite her marriage and move, she still wanted to be buried next to her first husband.

She thought she was crazy; but when she told me her story in 1975, I suggested that her night terror reflected a complicated and unfinished grief work. On the one hand, the dream had the features of a normal bereavement dream but indicated an unsatisfied need for attachment with the deceased. On the other hand, the terrifying presence, with its absence of distinct form, implies that the death has not been integrated into self-consciousness. The ambivalent absence and presence, desire and fear manifest on-going conflict in the relationship.

Underlying this ambivalence were two dynamic forces. One was a clinging to the deceased, a futile hanging on to him which created the ambivalence (Szondi 1980, 263). The other was a chronic guilt, probably due to the fact that she never encouraged her first husband to remove the shrapnel from his chest. Thus, a guilt-laden, agitated depression informed her background self, and, meanwhile, in the foreground she adapted to social reality by sustaining family life and working as a secretary.

She accepted my explanation of unfinished grief work, and, by gaining this insight, the presence ceased its regular visitations. However, the vision did not disappear entirely, but would reappear under two conditions. One, if her first son, having grown up and married, would come home for a visit, as on a holiday; and the other, when she would exchange emotion with him by letter or telephone. In either case, the presence would come precisely on the night before his visit or on the night after the emotional exchange. These two conditions imply that she was sustaining the bond with the first husband through the son.

This case demonstrates that night terrors, seemingly supernatural forces, derive from human relationships. The intensity of threat presupposes a distance in the relationship; for as one gets closer to death, anxiety diminishes. Since the relationship is impaired by chronic grieving, then the startle pattern is activated phobically. Normally, the consoling presence of dreams and visions suppresses the startle and comforts the bereaved. However, the night terror reveals a personal splitting, in which the ego, bereft of wholeness, submits to the intrusive force and wishes to die. The night terror frustrates the need for restitution, so that this need can only be satisfied in death.

V. HAUNTINGS AND RADIANT APPARITIONS

Occasionally, night terrors overlap with hauntings, which are exterior energy forces, acting intentionally, and appearing in a specific place, either for a short or long duration. Frederic Myers conceived of hauntings as "split-off" parts of a veridical afterimage. With the establishment of psychoanalysis, hauntings would be interpreted as projections of repressed or forbidden wishes by persons having low tolerance for frustration (Kastenbaum 1984, 124).

Some common hauntings are footsteps in the hallway, shuffling sounds, loud noises, opening doors, rocking chairs, luminous "ghosts," and the moving of bed covers. Less common would be enhanced scent from flowers. A former student describes her grandmother's terminal cancer:

> My grandmother had received these beautiful baby tea roses from a friend. And they were set on a table near where my grandmother was lying in her bed. And my grandfather had told my mom and aunts that every time he would enter the room and would go between the roses and my grandmother the scent was so strong. My mom told me that she can remember him describing it as a "scented path." This "scented path" was a direct path from the roses to my grandmother.

The scent expresses the shock of anticipatory grief, in as much as the sense of smell is a paroxysmal-epileptiform motif, as stated in chapter two.

Frequently, hauntings emanate from shock deaths, such as suicides and homicides, when restitution cannot be met. Marie-Louise von Franz theorizes that emotional intensities of death involve a struggle between bodily based affect and pure psychic energy escaping the body. The trauma of dying itself intensifies the psyche which, in the internal bodily struggle, expels affects explosively. She offers an example:

> When I was about twenty-four years old, I lived in a rented room in the house of a sixteen year old girl and her nurse. One night I dreamed that a terrible explosion occurred. The nurse and I crouched behind a wall in order not to be hit by stones and lumps of earth flying about. When I awakened I was informed

that during the night the girl had committed suicide with sleeping pills (von Franz 1987, 84).

She explains that with suicide the life energy is not used up naturally, and in the danger the archetype of fire takes over the energy. As argued in chapter two, fire symbolizes pent-up emotion, which is discharged to satisfy the need for restitution. With a suicide restitution cannot be made in life but only in death. Experimental data confirm that affective energy may be experienced telepathically in dreams (Ullman and Krippner 1973).

In her study of apparitions Aniela Jaffè has generalized on a wide range of case material and arrived at useful conclusions. When the dead are manifest apparitionally to relatives or close friends, they appear radiant and transfigured by a sublime beauty. Unrelated, deceased beings are disclosed as anonymous, veiled, shadowy, grey, or dark presences (Jaffè 1963, 56-57). Radiance denotes familial relatedness or friendship, and radiant apparitions in the veridical afterimage facilitate or help complete grief work. For example, a deceased father appeared to his daughter, several years after his death. He had died, when she was nine years old, and she grieved inconsolably for many years. One night on Christmas eve,

> suddenly I heard the door open and there were soft footsteps with a strange noise of knocking—I was alone at home and was rather frightened. Then the miracle happened—my beloved father came towards me, shining and lovely as gold, and transparent as mist. He looked just as he did in life, I could recognize his features quite clearly, then he stopped beside my bed and looked at me lovingly and smiled. A great peace entered into me and I felt happier than I had felt before...then he went away....(57)

VI. PROJECTIVE SHOCK VISIONS

On January 26, 1983 a former student of mine, then a social worker, discussed with me one of her current cases. A 25 year old musician was grieving the death of his wife in a brutal automobile accident. Two young children survived the death of their mother, and one child was a six month old baby boy. The man had frequent flashbacks to the scene of the accident during the day, and at night he often awakened with a startle. After awakening, he would behold his wife standing at the foot of the bed. He would separate from his body, float up to the ceiling and look back upon his body in bed, while his wife was calling to him. He would cry out to his parents, sleeping in the other room, to come and see that his wife had returned. She would say no and explained that she only wished to talk to him.

These visions took place during the first six months after the accident. Throughout that period, the baby slept in the same bed with his father; he too would awaken startled, as did his father, and he may have been aware of his mother standing at the foot of the bed. With the coming of the vision the man would feel fear and exhilaration. He wanted to go with her, but he had to stay with his children.

This case is unique with the combination of a "take-away" vision, "out-of-body" state, and symptoms of acute grief. The cycle of daily flashbacks and nightly startle conveys an intensity of grief with a deep sense of anxiety. The fear and exhilaration comprise the ambivalence that is characteristic of early grief. The flashbacks are an ad hoc introjection (*Augenblick-Introjektion*), which recollects the accident with an underlying guilt and depression. The flashback functions as a "possession-ideal" (*Besitzideale*), which triggers a desire to have the lost love object (Szondi 1956, 199). This desire is a motivating factor in the "out-of-body" phase of the grief. The bereaved man strips away his body, expands his psyche, in order to have his wife again. Thus, amid the ambivalent character of early grief work introjective and projective thought modes interact on a paroxysmal-hysteriform base. Both introjective and projective modes operate as defenses against death anxiety.

In the same year Elisabeth Kübler-Ross reported a similar situation, in which grief work was completed. A man suffered the death of his wife and children, who were burned to death in a fiery explosion, when their car was hit by a gasoline truck. Unable to resolve this tragedy, the man lost his job and home, became suicidal and addicted to cocaine, heroin, codeine, and vodka, in a desperate attempt to evade the grief. At one point in his despair, when drugged and drunk on a country road, he saw a large truck approaching:

> He watched, half-conscious, as the truck drove over him. He then became aware of drifting out of his body without any pain

or anxiety. He floated away and approached a light. Suddenly out of this light came his family! His wife and his children—as happy, healthy, and smiling as he remembered them, all of them together. "They did not speak, but I was able to understand everything. I suddenly knew that they were well. They had no scars, no burn marks. They were just there to show that they were all right and together" (Kübler-Ross 1983, 212).

He decided not to join them in death but willed to atone for his losses by achieving a constructive life.

The loss of his wife and the loss of his children created a two-fold grieving process. Parental loss of a child complicates grief work severely. The child is an extension of oneself, so that it is difficult to achieve detachment from the lost object. Such a loss inflicts a deep narcissistic wound, involving extreme ego phases. Thus, the grief was blocked by a total despair and negativism, as exemplified by suicide and addiction. These were inadequate forms of substitutionary participation with the dead. His shock on the country road stripped away his body and expanded his psyche to the point of a momentary participation. The vision of his family had the characteristics of a normal bereavement dream as well as those of a near-death experience. The projective-participatory shock vision resolved the despair, released his will to act, and provided a joyous atonement. The scenery of the vision (*seelische Schauplatz*) came out of the familial unconscious, which is the origin of the man's decision-making ability.

CHAPTER SIX:
ECSTASY OF MORTAL DANGER

I. ACCELERATION OF THOUGHT

The foregoing study of death-bed visions and bereavement dreams has shown that the shock of death generates a radiant being, which facilitates acceptance or participation, particularly in familial relationships. In this chapter our study extends to those cases, in which people have come close to death by trauma or by disease, survived and have been changed in some way. In his work Frederic Myers cited a case of apparent death and urged others to study this kind of situation (1903/1954, II, 315).

The principal theorist in modern times was Albert Heim, Professor of Geology at the University of Zürich, who was born in 1849 and died in 1937. Professionally, he conducted research on the structure of the Alps and, in the course of his work, suffered several falls. He reflected on his own falls and studied those of thirty other persons. In 1892 he published a paper analyzing the impact of the falls, and it has been translated into English by Russell Noyes and Roy Kletti with the title "Remarks on Fatal Falls" (1972, 45-52).

Heim discovered that 95% of fall victims had the same kind of experience, regardless of the nature of their mishap, and he summarized the uniform core as follows:

> ...no grief was felt, nor was there paralyzing fright of the sort that can happen in instances of lesser danger (e.g. outbreak of fire). There was no anxiety, no trace of despair, no pain, but rather calm seriousness, profound acceptance, and a dominant mental quickness and sense of surety, mental activity became

enormous, rising to a hundred-fold velocity or intensity. The relationships of events and their probable outcomes were overviewed with objective clarity. No confusion entered at all. Time became greatly expanded. The individual acted with lightning-quickness in accord with accurate judgment of his situation (46-47).

Heim added that in some cases there may be a life review, the hearing of beautiful celestial music, or a transfiguration by light.

During the crisis, victims act consciously and not reflexively. The impact of the shock reveals a natural necessity to which they surrender. Giving into the necessity evokes love, harmony, and fusion of subject and object. In the face of death conflict dissolves. However, should any illness be present already, then the victim's consciousness may be clouded.

Heim achieved a fundamental insight, namely, that in the most profound startle the mind accelerates rapidly, achieving active control without pain. In contrast, superficial surprises result in a paralysis of thought and action. Thus, dread exhibits a distance from the object or from the danger. Heim's insights imply that mind varies with respect to the intensity of shock. Both high and low level threats presuppose a permeable continuum of paroxysmal activity. To be close to death is to be less threatened, to be distanced more so.

Paralysis also comes to those who witness fatal or near fatal accidents. From the outside the trauma seems horrible and has long-lasting effects; but from the inside the trauma delivers the victim into an intensely pleasurable state.

In the absence of preceding illness it ensues in clear consciousness, in heightened sensory and ideational activity, and without anxiety or pain. Those of our friends who have died in the mountains have, in their last moments, reviewed their individual pasts in states of transfiguration (51).

Enhanced peace, joy, and painlessness are psychic equivalents of death. Although Heim's paper contained seminal insights, it was essentially neglected until 1930, when Oskar Pfister published a psychoanalytic analysis of his findings. Pfister's paper has been translated into English by Noyes and Kletti with the title "Shock Thoughts and Fantasies in

Extreme Mortal Danger" (1981, 5-20). Pfister acknowledges that in moments of danger thought speeds up or slows down, but he wonders which occurs under what conditions. After reading Heim's paper, Pfister points out that shock-thought is determined by two activities. One is reality based, and the other is an autistic denial of the shock itself. The denial derives from the intensification of thought, exclusion of fear, and pleasurable fantasies. Since Pfister himself had fallen twice in the mountains, he asserts that the "fall and its danger are first realized, then derealized."

Previously, Pfister had written a letter to Heim, inquiring about his personal fall experiences. Heim replied in a letter on December 17, 1929, which Pfister quoted in his paper. Several lines are excerpted below:

> In the moment in which I slipped in a difficult place it was clear to me that I would fall helplessly and quite probably to my death. This quick insight produced, however, no fright, no anxiety.
>
> I then had a series of singularly clear flashes of thought among a rapid, profuse succession of images that were clear and distinct. Thoughtful recollections were mixed with exhilarating representations, perhaps also hallucinations. I couldn't say what the exact succession was. I believe that it was almost instantaneous. I can perhaps compare it best to rapidly projected images or with the rapid sequence of dream images.
>
> I saw the images as though they were projected on a wall. One gave way to another, but all without haste, in a pleasing sequence and with copious changings, without any emotional interruptions.
>
> I acted out my life, as though I were an actor on a stage, upon which I looked down as though from practically the highest gallery in the theatre. Both hero and onlooker, I was as though doubled.
>
> My sisters and especially my wonderful mother, who was so important in my life, were around me.
>
> It was a feeling of submission to necessity. There I was arching over me...a beautiful blue sky.... There sounded solemn music.... It seems that the theatrical performance of my life

began with school and ended with the fall backwards into emptiness or sky (9-10).

Pfister defines Heim's images as autistic fantasies that "replace and repress" thought about physical reality. The principle is the same as that in dreamwork; "To protect us from shock, the unconscious occupies us with fantasy, manufacturing it from emotionally comforting images that are meaningless because [it is] torn out of context" (12). From Heim's experiences, Pfister deduces the following defenses against the threat of mortal danger; (1) replacing disturbing content with non-threatening material; (2) defending against danger by making it delusional or weakened, as with *deja vu*; (3) admitting pain but without details; and (4) overcoming of dread by comforting and pleasing fantasy (13).

Pfister takes over Freud's concept of the stimulus barrier, which means that the mind pervades the entire sensory system, defending against threats in accord with the pleasure principle. With reference to mortal danger the pleasure principle generates shock fantasies as forms of defense. Pfister also confirms Heim's insights into the degrees of shock but explains that the observed acceleration of thought is actually a separation from reality through derealization, which "is like the feeling of being a mere spectator and seeing one's life passing across a stage" (14). Derealization resembles splitting, even though the identity of the observer remains intact.

Pfister acknowledges different kinds of shock fantasies that transform reality. Some project comforting memories, others those of the future, metaphysical places, celestial music, or religious beliefs. These are like day dreams in the sense that they protect waking consciousness and prevent sleeping or fainting. In contrast, dreams protect sleep by allowing the sleeper to enjoy wish-fulfilling images. Both dreams and shock fantasies are regressive, because the life review presents only the pleasurable moments of one's past and not one's entire life. The *deja vu* diminishes danger by giving the victim the impression of having been through the crisis previously. The pleasure principle triumphs over the reality principle through the absence of pain and the displacement of death by childhood wishes.

When the threat of death invades the sensory systems, pleasurable fantasies erupt like a flash into consciousness from the unconscious. Fantasies are projected by the unconscious will to live, and the flash is released by the preconscious, acting as a filter between consciousness and unconsciousness. Shock fantasies totally dominate consciousness, expelling any awareness of death.

In conclusion, the principal value of Pfister's paper is his preserving Heim's original findings; otherwise, he succeeds only in presenting a questionable interpretation, because Freud's theory of mind has been challenged by neurology. In the remainder of this section I sketch an interpretation of Heim's findings which are summarized as follows: (1) acceleration of thought; (2) reduction of pain and anxiety; (3) consciousness of death; (4) projected imagery and duality of observer and observed; (5) submission to necessity; and (6) aura of emptiness.

The intense acceleration of thought indicates adaptation to mortal danger and a turning toward fundamental reality. The turn takes place in the submission to necessity. Within fundamental reality time and space are relativized, and personal being is transformed into pure form without matter, extension or continuum. The reduction of pain and anxiety presupposes the annulment of the startle pattern and an opening onto a transcendent reality. Since pain varies with cortical levels, its reduction reveals the hierarchical organization of the brain. Higher meanings nullify the pain messages of the sensory systems. With its complexity the mind can adapt to life-threatening crises without regressing. Adaptation is aided by dreamwork, which functions to generate meaning and value and not just to protect sleep. Adaptation also includes knowledge of death, and this facilitates transcendent meaning and value.

The work of projection in the ego is to activate the primal drive for participation in metaphysical reality. Projection is a normal function of a healthy mind. The duality of observer and observed conforms to Szondi's participatory theory of dreamwork, advanced in chapter four. Observing does not mean splitting or derealizing; rather it signifies the receding of waking consciousness, when it surpasses a threshold and becomes hypnagogic. At this point the background self comes out in the form of unconscious personal, familial, and archetypal content. Frequently, the life review unfolds on the stage of the psyche prompting choices or submission to necessity. Finally, the "aura of emptiness" means that the self has become hypnopompic by means of epileptiform seizure activity. The Heim aura is like the Dostoevsky aura, with its sublime feelings of peace, joy, painlessness, and harmony. The seizure coincides with the shock of mortal danger and the resulting aura is both defensive and participatory. The sense of emptiness is not derealization but an adaptive fulfillment of the drive for participation. The aura of emptiness actualizes pontifical selfhood.

II. THE DEATH-FEIGNING REFLEX

In current discussions the tradition of Heim and Pfister is carried on by Russell Noyes, who not only confirms Heim's findings but also accounts for them by the concept of depersonalization. Noyes draws upon the work of Martin Roth and Max Harper, who claim that depersonalization informs both epilepsy and phobic anxiety (1962). They treat epilepsy as a purely neurological disturbance and neurosis as purely emotional, involving mainly phobic and avoidance reactions. Their approach goes against the neuropsychiatric perspective, stated in chapter one, according to which epilepsy has both neural and emotional aspects and neuroses derive from specific genetic groups.

Roth and Harper define depersonalization as "that dissociation or duplication of consciousness which is particularly associated with any heightening of stimulation that evokes acute fear or anxiety" (219). When confronting danger, depersonalization helps one to survive through vigilance and detachment. However, under extreme conditions normal adaptation may become exaggerated by inducing a "phobic-anxiety depersonalization syndrome," which manifests a "jerky, overresponsiveness...irritability, restlessness, insomnia," with closed-eye hallucinations if awake or hypnagogic hallucinations if falling asleep. In a neurosis energy overflows in the forms of traumas, palpitations, excessive perspiration, intolerance of heat, and attacks of panic. Hence, neurosis is a maladaptive variant of adaptive vigilance.

With the data offered by Roth and Harper Noyes claims to have discovered a neural mechanism, which is activated in times of danger. The mechanism responds to perilous stimuli in alternating modes: heightened arousal, on the one hand, and dissociation of consciousness (depersonalization), on the other (Noyes 1979, 78). The former enhances vigilance, and the latter reduces potentially disorganizing consciousness. In either case, anxiety is present.

Noyes makes depersonalization a psychological defense against death. To be depersonalized is to mimic death, becoming numb, empty, and lifeless so as not be threatened. In the mimicry the ego splits into an observing self, separated from the threat in order to survive. The other part of the ego, the observed and embodied self, is sacrificed as it takes the brunt of the shock. Altogether the splitting is characterized by separation from the body, loss of emotion, altered sense of time, derealization of the physical world, and alien sights and sounds. These traits are obtained from falls, automobile accidents, near-drownings, cardiac arrests, combat explosions, and allergic reactions.

As a polar mechanism, depersonalization adapts to two kinds of danger. First, if one perceives impending death but does not actually die, then one experiences hyperalertness, including accelerated thought, enhanced seeing and hearing, altered sense of time, feeling of bliss, and possibly a life review. This hyperalertness-depersonalization would supposedly account for Heim's findings.

Second, if one actually dies and is resuscitated, then one enters a mystical state. Mystical-depersonalization goes beyond a psychological defense to a genuinely spiritual dimension. It brings deep feelings of knowledge, clear images and visions, derealization of the body, recollections, control by outside forces, and revelation of joy and harmony. An example of this mystical harmony comes from a soldier whose jeep was blown up by a Nazi mine in World War II:

> Almost immediately after the explosion, I was certain that death had occurred. I experienced no physical sensations, no sense perceptions. Rather I seemed to have entered a state in which only my thoughts or mind existed. I felt total serenity and peace. I had no remembrance of anything, only a realization that life had ended and that my mind was continuing to exist. I had no realization of time passing, only of one moment which never altered. Neither did I have any concept of space, since my existence seemed only mental. I cannot stress strongly enough the feeling of total peace of mind and of total blissful acceptance of my new status, which I knew would be never ending (Noyes and Kletti 1982, 61).

This mystical-depersonalization may unfold in three stages: (1) The impact of death evokes alarm, followed by resistance, fear, or struggle; then an upsurge of life energy that is blocked by an urge to surrender. (2) Having lost control, one beholds the life review as a panoramic replay of positive biographical events, when the observing self splits off from the body. (3) One enters a transcendent state of ecstasy, which is ineffable, timeless, spaceless, and unified, disclosing ultimate truth (Noyes 1972, 179-180).

Noyes' theory goes beyond Pfister's by properly emphasizing that the mind adapts to extreme danger and does not regress. Noyes is more coherent in the sense that he respects the complex unity of the brain-mind system and displays more precision in search of a neural location for the experience. He also acknowledges the limitations of scientific method, when he accepts a mystical and religious dimension.

Nevertheless, I believe he appeals to a questionable model of epilepsy, and so I offer a critical assessment of Noyes' position. An even more coherent explanation may be gained by recognizing that epilepsy and phobic anxiety, mimicry and mystical ecstasy are polar eruptions of the paroxysmal pattern. As conceptualized by Szondi, the paroxysmal pattern shares a genetic homology with the "feigning-death reflex" (*Totstellreflex*), which is a phylogenetic defense against danger that immobilizes oneself so as to appear dead (1960, 113). For humans the same reflex informs the clinical fact that epilepsy mimics or substitutes for death. The paroxysmal pattern also accounts for the acceleration of thought in the midst of danger, which yields a sense of ecstasy.

The paroxysmal pattern unfolds in a three fold rhythm: (1) accumulation of affect; (2) explosive discharge of affect, making one lose control and become unconscious; and (3) movement toward restitution or even the mystical ecstasy. This model may be considered as the motor-force behind Noyes' three fold scheme of mystical experience: (1) alarm, resistance, struggle; (2) life review; and (3) transcendence.

In my view, depersonalization is the wrong term, because, as Noyes himself says, it narrows attention, reduces feeling, and causes a dullness or numbing (Noyes and Kletti 1982, 62). Depersonalized people become estranged from themselves, lifeless automatons and seemingly dead. They neither feel anything nor recall memories. When compared to epilepsy, depersonalization may come after or between seizures, but it certainly does not fit the Dostoevsky aura. Both Heim and Noyes describe profound joy and ecstasy at the brink of death, but these are not a depersonalization.

Depersonalization is essentially a psychotic state, in which all perceptions and feelings are destroyed (Szondi 1977, 326-327). In contrast, the shock of mortal danger instigates the startle and then, by means of accelerated thought, generates a psychic intensity co-existing with diminishing spatio-temporal forms. The intensification of thought and feeling causes the waking consciousness to recede, while the primal drive for participation emerges from the unconscious. Paroxysmal-participation rather than depersonalization coheres with Noyes' findings as well as Heim's.

III. DESTINY AND THE PRIMAL FORM

In 1944 Carl Jung suffered a heart attack, and he wrote in his autobiography that he "hung on the edge of death and was being given oxygen and camphor injections" (1961, 289). After recovering, his nurse told him that a bright glow had emanated from him, while clinically dead. Jung said that he had floated up into space:

Far below I saw the globe of the earth, bathed in a glorious blue light. I saw the deep blue sea and the continents. Far below my feet lay Ceylon, and in the distance ahead of me the subcontinent of India. My field of vision did not include the whole earth, but its global shape was plainly distinguishable and its outline shone with a silvery gleam through that wonderful blue light (289).

Jung entered a temple through a dark chamber and felt that his entire bodily existence was being stripped away in a painful process, leaving the basic core of his life:

This experience gave me a feeling of extreme poverty, but at the same time of great fullness. There was no longer anything I wanted or desired. I existed in an objective form; I was what I had been and lived. At first the sense of annihilation predominated, of having been stripped or pillaged; but suddenly that became of no consequence (291).

Jung considered his life to be a fragment, an excerpt from a story, without beginning and without end. While floating in space, he saw the universe as an artificially constructed three-dimensional box.

From the direction of Europe the image of his physician floated up and delivered a message. He, that is, Jung had to return to earth. Jung resisted the return and, at the same time, worried about his doctor; for once one attains primal form, one must die. The doctor did die a few days after Jung's recovery, but no explanation is given as to why Jung survived, assuming he also attained his primal form.

In the days following his resuscitation Jung alternated between waking and dream consciousness. In his "split-off" phase he floated again into the emptiness of the universe and felt a profound ecstasy. His feelings of beauty were the most intense he had ever experienced, "utterly real; there was nothing subjective about them; they all had a quality of absolute objectivity" (295). He portrays his vision as "the ecstasy of a non-temporal state in which present, past, and future are one." Nothing fit into an extensive continuum; everything was one and whole. Jung means individuation or self-realization, which is finished in death. His self-realization was symbolized by his beholding the heavenly wedding in the garden of pomegranates, in Jerusalem, and in a classical amphitheatre at the end of a valley surrounded by hills.

Sometime later, Jung wrote in a letter that, during his illness whatever "you do, if you do it sincerely, will eventually become the bridge to your wholeness, a good ship that carries you through the darkness of your second birth, which seems to be death to the outside" (1973, 358-359). Here Jung affirms his primal form with the symbol of the bridge.

Two months before his death on June 6, 1961, Jung dreamed of arriving in Bollingen made of gold. Bollingen was the name of the tower that Jung built beside Lake Zürich; he began construction in 1923, the year of his mother's death, and completed it in 1955, the year of his wife's death. Building Bollingen was a part of Jung's grief work. So in the dream, two months before his own death, Jung "held the key to the tower in his hand and a voice told him that the 'tower' was now completed and ready for habitation" (cited in von Franz 1987, 130). This dream reflected the dream he had immediately after completing the tower, in which he saw a replica of the tower standing on the distant shore of the lake.

Taken together, Jung's vision and related dreams clearly illustrate projection and symbolism of shock events. The stripping away of his bodily existence was the start of his projective-participatory mode of being. The strength of the "stripping" might be genotropic, since Jung's biography gives evidence of projective, even schizoform factors. For example, he was a psychiatrist, his maternal grandmother a spiritualist medium, his first cousin a medium, the maternal grandfather a physician and professor, all of which indicating a hereditary tendency toward projective expansiveness in decision-making. The ecstasy of the non-temporal state, which he attained, manifests the exaltation of the power of being and pontifical selfhood, as represented himself by the bridge symbol. His participatory state grew out of the shock of the heart attack and exhibited paroxysmal symbolic motifs, such as "floating" high up in space (air), beholding light (fire), seeing the subcontinent of India (earth), and the deep blue sea (water). When he achieved his primal being, he saw his life as a thread of destiny, which is the function of the life review, and the revelation of his destiny took shape as a primal necessity.

IV. ANALYSIS OF THE CORE NDE

In the generation following the death of Carl Jung his vision came to be known as a near-death experience. This well-known term, designated NDE, was developed in a popular book by Raymond Moody, who studied 150 near-death cases (1975). That a new term had to be created meant that the classical heritage of visions, which Jung represented, had either been unknown or lost to contemporary American society. After his initial publication, Moody published a more extensive study, based upon one thousand cases, that established the core traits of the NDE: (1) sense of being dead; (2) painless peace despite "painful" experience; (3) bodily separation; (4) entrance into a dark region; (5) rapid rise to the heavens; (6) meeting deceased friends or relatives bathed in light; and (7) encountering a Supreme Being; (8) the life review; and (9) reluctance to return (1988, 2). These characteristics are taken from accidents, resuscitations from clinical death, and other traumas, such as nonfatal suicide attempts. Moody suggests that one or more of these experiences constitute the NDE.

Moody emphasizes that NDE survivors feel love and peace, lose a fear of death, and gain a new appreciation of knowledge as well as a deeper spirituality. Ironically, with greater wisdom and deeper feeling they may have difficulty interacting with the ordinary social world, following their return from death or unconsciousness. Their difficulty derives from the fact that, while clinically dead, they had "separated" from their physical bodies and discovered a new spiritual "body," in which they became whole, mobile, and complete. The spiritual "body" has neither defect nor handicap. Similarly, Elisabeth Kübler-Ross adds that "amputees had their legs again, those who were in wheelchairs could dance and move around without any effort, and blind people could see" (1983, 208).

Moody goes on to say that a Supreme Being is encountered as a Being of Light, which is intense but nonthreatening. Nonverbal communication in the form of telepathy takes place between the Being of Light and the person in the spiritual "body" (Moody 1988, 12). Telepathy entails a dimension of thought existing independently of sensory-muscular systems. Other investigators support this claim on the grounds that knowledge increases as brain activity decreases and, therefore, discloses a transcendental source beyond psychological and physiological causes (Owens, et. al. 1990). Further, a study of the transforming effects of NDEs, over a span of ten years, finds decreased death anxiety, increased psychic ability, zest for life, and a higher level of intelligence (Morse with Perry 1992, 58-59).

Moody also identifies a life review, which tends to unfold as a third person, three-dimensional, full color panorama. The Being of Light presents the life review, which contains the consequences of the actions committed in one's life, including shameful and evil deeds. The encounter with the Being of Light usually comes after one floats through a long, dark tunnel in the disembodied or spiritual state. As long as one occupies the spiritual "body," one displays a flow pattern of form and energy, in which time is compressed and spatial boundaries surpassed.

To compare the Moody-type NDE with the classical models of Heim and Jung would demonstrate a basic convergence. Moody's discovery of a rapid ascent, telepathy, relativization of space-time, and Being of Light presupposes an acceleration of thought. Throughout NDE accounts acceleration occurs in the out-of-body state, as illustrated in a description of a cardiac arrest:

> Almost immediately I saw myself leave my body, coming out through my head and shoulders (I did not see my lower limbs). The "body" leaving me was not exactly in vapour form, yet it seemed to expand very slightly once it was clear of me. It was somewhat transparent, for I could see my other "body" through it.
>
> Suddenly I am sitting on a very small object travelling at great speed, out and up into a dull blue-grey sky, at a 45-degree angle (MacMillan and Brown 1982, 48).

However, unlike Jung, Heim and Moody's patients discovered deceased relatives in the NDEs. Jung failed to clarify the distinctive familial dimension of the unconscious, and, consequently, clinicians who follow him employ an incomplete model of the unconscious. Since the familial unconscious is omitted in the NDE literature, investigators conceive of deceased relatives as actual entities, whose postmortem existence proves life after death. This seems to be Moody's position, and, as an example, one of his subjects says that, during a difficult labor, she

> lost consciousness, and heard an annoying buzzing, ringing sound. The next thing I knew it seemed as if I were on a ship or a small vessel sailing to the other side of a large body of water. On the distant shore, I could see all of my loved ones who had died--my mother, my father, my sister, and others. I could see them, could see their faces, just as they were when I knew them on earth. They seemed to be beckoning me to come on over, and all the while I was saying, "no, no, I'm not ready to go" (1975, 74-75).

I interpret the noise in the head as an epileptiform seizure, as would Moody but in another context (1975, 140). The water is a paroxysmal shock symbol, and the sailing is the cross-over archetype. Meeting relatives is the same as encountering their forms in the familial unconscious. The key element is the woman's decision to return, a factor consistent with the familial origin of decision-making.

The issue of the unconscious was raised by Michael Sabom who, when assessing Moody's data, insisted that no medical model of the unconscious had yet been proposed as a verifiable concept (1982, 7). Sabom conceives of the unconscious as a period of time wherein the person loses all subjective awareness of self and environment. This notion closely resembles that of clinical death, a state in which all external signs of consciousness, reflexes, respiration, and cardiac activity are absent, but the organism is not fully dead. Without any medical intervention, within five or six minutes, the organism will proceed on a natural course toward biological death, which is the total and irreversible cessation of all metabolic activity. Under certain conditions clinical death is reversible.

Sabom essentially confirmed Moody's findings, and he emphasized that with separation from the physical body one becomes an essential self, invisible and nonmaterial. One goes into an autoscopic phase with a sense of timelessness, reality, and death; feelings of peace; and absence of pain. A unique capacity of the essential self is a striking clarity of thought, characterized by acceleration. One subject recalls:

> I could have moved away from my body anytime I wanted to....
> There wasn't a thing that was mechanical about it, like an automobile or anything. It was just a thought process. I felt like I could have thought myself anywhere I wanted to be instantly....
> I just felt exhilarated with a sense of power (Sabom 1982, 34).

Some of Sabom's subjects went from an earthly environment to a transcendent realm through a dark region or void toward light. In the transcendent region they encounter nonvisual presences or visualized spirits, who are deceased relatives or religious figures, with whom verbal, nonverbal, telepathic, or gestural communication takes place. A life review may occur, usually early in the process, prior to a full loss of consciousness (50). The NDE ends with a return to the body, after one has reached a limit.

Sabom's work is analytic and carefully crafted, but the question arises: Is the loss of subjective awareness sufficient for the acquisition of the transcendental experiences? I believe Sabom's data would become more coherent, if his "negative" model of the unconscious were replaced by the tripartite view proposed in chapter two. Nonvisual presences or deceased relatives would emanate from the familial unconscious, and visualized spirits the collective. Telepathy presumes an expansion of mind beyond the subjective ego and participation in a transpersonal relatedness. Likewise, the life review presupposes the retention of one's actions in an unconscious dimension which exists independently of the vital signs.

Failure of researchers to acknowledge a complete view of the unconscious, particularly the familial, implies a preference for linear and sequential categories. Along with Sabom, Kenneth Ring is credited with verifying Moody's data. Ring sorted out the basic NDE characteristics into a statistically probable stage theory: (1) affective well-being; (2) separation from the body; (3) immersion in a dark void or tunnel; (4) seeing the light at the end of the tunnel and moving toward it; and (5) entering the light (1980, 67-68). Along the way, one could encounter the life review, deceased relatives, and Spiritual Being, before returning to bodily consciousness. Ring emphasizes that deceased relatives encourage the return, for the completion of responsibilities, for example; but the Spiritual Being offers one a choice of returning or not. In contrast, Moody has stated that choice or encouragement could come either from relatives or the Being of Light. Ring also amplifies the life review by adding a flash-forward, instead of a flash-back, precognitive, planetary, and prophetic visions, such as those of impending catastrophes, landmass changes, earthquakes, or war (1984, 183-192). Prophetic visions are rare; but when they happen, they disclose a scenario of cosmic necessity and regeneration.

Ring's stages are consecutive and invariant. His so-called "invariant hypothesis" has been challenged by Bruce Greyson, who posits four distinct categories: cognitive, affective, paranormal, and transcendental (1985, 968). He argues that the nature of the NDE shapes the functional type. For example, when death is not anticipated, as in an accident, then transcendental, affective and cognitive forms co-act with equal frequency. When death is anticipated, then affective and transcendental forms dominate. Thus, in the expected NDE, cognitive aspects are rare; and these include time distortion, acceleration of thought, and sudden understanding. The implication of Greyson's argument is that NDEs have diverse origins without consecutive stages.

When viewed together, Greyson's and Ring's theories pose a subject-object dichotomy, respectively. Greyson introduces a subjectivist bias, when making thought acceleration and time distortion cognitive features. Ring presumes the reality of the object in proposing a linear model. The emerging conclusion of this chapter is that thought acceleration derives from fundamental reality, in which subject-object, space-time forms are relativized. Disclosure of fundamental reality occurs in an epileptiform shock event, that dissolves such distinctions as cognition and affect.

V. NEGATIVE NDES

All investigators acknowledge that not everyone who comes close to death has the NDE. A recent study has estimated about 40-45% of persons have one (Brooks 1991, 22). Obviously, this raises questions about the other 60-55%. One explanation is that persons who do not go far enough toward death lack the NDE, because the experience is a memory, created "on the way back," by patients attempting to make sense of the crisis (Kastenbaum 1991, 323). Upon recovering, they are able to integrate the feelings with a narrative recollection. This argument presupposes the Freudian model of the psyche, according to which one recollects the trauma, overcomes resistance, and works it through with feelings and symbolic forms.

To explore this line of thought I draw upon a case study, conducted by one of my students, who is an experienced emergency medical paramedic. On the night of February 9, 1991, he was called to the home of a 26 year old, married woman, mother of two sons. She was "pale, breathless, and without a pulse," in a state of ventricular fibrillation, a form of clinical death. After defibrillation and intravenous treatment, she was taken to a hospital, where a defibrillation system was surgically implanted. Throughout the paramedic process, she received oxygen therapy.

When speaking with the woman later, the paramedic learned that she had no memory from one and one half days before the trauma until six or seven days after resuscitation. While in the hospital, family members observed swelling in her face. The paramedic interpreted the swelling to mean increased carbon dioxide and decreased oxygen levels. Since paramedics needed almost six minutes to reach her home, this cerebral anoxia might have blocked the short term memory.

Nevertheless, the victim has had a recurrent dream, coming regularly long after her cardiac arrest. She dreams of herself

> lying in a hospital bed with nurses and doctors around her. They appear to be talking to her; however, she is unable to interpret or respond back to them, while at the same time the nurses and doctors are performing acts of patient care.

The dream seems to be an accurate recollection of the hospital setting; yet when asked to recall what happened, she described darkness, loneliness, and an increased fear of death. Despite this negative image, she acquired a heightened spirituality and zest for life, which belong to NDEs. She began to work for the Ladies Auxiliary of the fire department, Little League World Series, and Head Start.

Except for her new intensity, this woman does not precisely exhibit the traits of the NDE. Psychoanalytically, the woman gets a narrative recollection "on the way back" but fails to work through the trauma, due to a persistent fear of death as darkness and loneliness. Instead of imposing a backward-forward sequential model, it would be more appropriate to make a threshold analysis, as with death-bed visions. The woman's recollection does not achieve wholeness, because she fails to resolve some type of conflict, probably in her family relationships.

So-called negative NDEs are reported in the literature occasionally, and, as an example, Robert Kastenbaum quotes one survivor of an automobile accident:

> I was thrilled to meet this person or was it an angel--and then all at once I saw that she or it was truly horrible. Where the eyes were supposed to be were slits and kind of blue-green flames flickered through them, through the eye-places. I can still see this demon, this whatever-it-was. With my eyes wide open, I can still see it (1991, 322).

A pioneering study describes negative NDEs as dominated by fear and anguish, with out-of-body states, movement through a dark tunnel or void, being of light, judgment of past deeds, and meeting deceased acquaintances. However, the movement through the tunnel has a downward trajectory, and the transcendent environment is hellish, dark, misty, with a cave or lake of fire, and demonic beings (Irwin and Bramwell 1988, 38-40).

To illustrate, the authors describe an automobile accident, in which the driver, a 50 year old woman, is lifted up to a high place and goes through a tunnel to a field of light. She sees a church in the distance; so she walks toward it and enters through the front door. Inside the sanctuary people are wearing black robes and red hoods. She advances toward the altar, on top of which stands a silver jug and six silver goblets.

> I stood there wondering where I was and what I was doing there, when a door opened to the right of the altar and out came the devil. He came over to the altar, looked me straight in the eye and told me to pick up a goblet. I picked up a goblet and he picked up the big silver jug and started pouring. I saw that what he was pouring from the jug was *fire*, and I screamed, dropped the goblet and started to run. I just ran and ran. I didn't know where I was running to. And then I saw a big fence, a stone

fence, and the gates opened and I passed through. Then I came to another fence made out of iron bars, and that just opened, and again I ran through. All the time I was getting warmer and warmer and brighter and brighter (42).

The experience ended, when she awakened in a hospital room.

These two cases exhibit fire, a figure of evil, and fear. The authors generalize from the second that the NDE is a holistic event with contrasting phases. They oppose the notion that different NDEs have diverse origins. In my view, they are correct, and their interpretation may be amplified by reconsidering paroxysmal symbolism. Fire represents pent-up Cain affects, and the devil archetype indicates that the anger, rage or resentment lack restitution. Running away is a hysteroid reaction, a fear growing out of the pent-up anger, and the opening of the doors is an attempt to work the anger through the hierarchical layers of the brain-mind system. Getting warmer and warmer means the build up of the affect to an epileptiform seizure. In both cases pent-up emotion indicates unresolved conflict and the failure to achieve integration, transcendence, and participation.

VI. PEDIATRIC NDES

The current search to understand NDEs includes those of children, who are relatively free of cultural conditioning and who offer the possibility of a pure experience. Generally, pediatric NDEs are like those of adults, except that they omit a life review due to their short life span. Children tend to discover loving beings, specifically next of kin, who have preceded them in death.

One child who was almost lost during very critical heart surgery shared with her father that she was met by a brother with whom she felt so comfortable; it was as if they had known each other and shared each other's lives. Yet, she had never had a brother. Her father was very moved by his daughter's account and confesses that she did have a brother, but he had died before she was born (Kübler-Ross, 1983, 208).

This case illustrates how the NDE penetrates the familial unconscious, existing at a deeper level than the personal unconscious.

The familial unconscious is the medium through which siblings are reciprocally attracted to each other by means of genotropism. Genotropism operates in the death state by virtue of the fact that relationships survive death and are preserved unconsciously in the family.

The case material even includes family pets in the pediatric NDEs. One investigator describes the drowning of an eight year old boy, who separates from his body and proceeds through a tunnel toward a light. He has no life review, and time stops in the tunnel. He turns right and discovers two family pets: a springer spaniel, who had died when the boy was three, and a deceased cat. They lick the boy's face, and then he pets them (Serdahely 1989-1990, 59). The NDE ends, when the boy awakens in a hospital.

In a subsequent publication the same investigator reports the case of a young girl, clinically dead for thirty seconds. She enters a dark region in a peaceful, painless state, when a lamb approaches, comes close, and then runs away (Serdahely 1990, 249-250). The lamb had also been a deceased pet.

Psychoanalysts would interpret these encounters in terms of transference. The Being of Light is a transference of the love of the father in a protective manner. The transference satisfies the need to deny death and allow the triumph of infantile omnipotence. In the two cases cited above the pets substitute for the parents, but the projected need remains the same. Further, the out-of-body state is an uncoupling of the mental ego from the bodily ego. The former splits off and observes the latter (Gabbard and Twemlow 1984, 160, 238). This position rests upon a philosophical monism, according to which the physical and psychological processes are identical. Hence, the so-called splitting of the egoes is only a matter of perspective and not a real separation, because nothing exists outside the brain.

However, the author of the pet studies reports that the mother of the eight year old boy had a premonition of his fall and that throughout his unconscious state, she spoke to him in a loving manner. Her premonition posits clairvoyance at a distance with translocal and transcausal relatedness. Since the boy could hear his mother and his father speaking, while unconscious, he maintained a level of awareness independent of the comatose brain. These facts refute a monism and require a transpersonal state of being with a reciprocal family participation.

Meeting deceased pets indicates that the death state activates the need for attachment. Pets are familiar beings and, as such, belong to the background self. Szondi defines the background self psychologically and biologically, but he does not restrict it to the same species (1977, 234). As long as pets satisfy the need for attachment through contact-bonding, then their relatedness could be preserved unconsciously. The decisive insight of the pet cases is that instinctual drive material operates during clinical death. Szondi derives the need for attachment from the contact drive (1963, 479).

A definitive analysis of childhood NDEs comes out of the work of Melvin Morse. He conducted a study of 121 children, who were intubated or attached to artificial lung machines, thus ruling out anoxia as a cause. Nearly all of his children, as well as 25% of adults, see the light (Morse with Perry 1990, 115). Light normally appears after bodily separation and travel through the tunnel. The light is a warm, caring, wrap-around presence that is not confined to the boundaries of the body.

If the light were exclusively physiological and eyesight were to cease, Morse argues, then darkness ought to appear. Instead, light dawns in death, and so it cannot be derived from "spasm of rigor mortis in the optic nerve" (133). The light radiates life-giving, transforming qualities, and it even extends beyond the physical boundaries of the body. Thus, light cannot be reduced psychoanalytically to a transference of the father's love.

Morse describes a child, who fell overboard from a boat into the dark murky waters of Puget Sound in Washington. Her father jumped into the water and made several surface dives in an attempt to recover her. Because the water was so dark, he could not see her. After diving unsuccessfully, he finally saw a light in the depths of the waters. He swam toward the light and saw that his daughter's limp body was emitting it. He grabbed her and took her to the surface, where she was rescued. Hence, at the point of death the light shone in the darkness of the waters.

Morse's cases reveal that the light takes a symbolic form, particularly the cross-over archetype. For example, six year old Daniel was hit by a car. He left his body, travelled down a dark tunnel to the light, where he saw three men, behind whom was "a rainbow bridge that stretched across the sky" (40). The boy did not go with the three men, because he wished to return to his parents.

Seven year old Cary was dying of leukemia. He moved up a beam of light to heaven, crossed over a rainbow bridge, and visited a crystal castle (53). God told him that he would die at a specific time, and this prediction turned out to be correct.

VII. EXPLANATIONS OF SEIZURES

One of the significant aspects of Morse's work is his claim to have discovered the neurological cause of the NDE. The right temporal lobe of the brain contains a genetically coded program for the NDE, which operates in the shock of mortal danger (100). In a subsequent study he explains that everything but the light may be located physiologically in the brain (Morse with Perry 1992, 67). The light shines only in death, and the energy of the light flows into the organism through the right temporal lobe, where it comes to a peak, releases energy, and even radiates outside the body. The build up and release of light through the organism causes the most profound transformations, including the clinically observed decrease of anxiety and increase of paranormal psychic ability, involving telepathy and precognitive dreams. Morse documents the fact that survivors of NDEs have four times as many psychic experiences as non-NDEers (89). Ironically, 25% of adult NDE survivors stop wearing watches, simply because they cease working (132). Morse speculates that discharge of light in the NDE changes the electromagnetic forces in the cells and body; and these energy forces effect the watches.

Morse's conclusion bears upon the modern scientific study of epilepsy; for to locate the NDE in the right temporal lobe is to establish a neurological relationship with temporal lobe epilepsy. Demonstrating that the light cannot be located means that the NDE opens up the brain to a transcendent reality. Morse's description of the build up and discharge of light parallels the accumulation and explosion of affect in temporal lobe epilepsy, including the Dostoevsky aura. The factor which connects the NDE and temporal lobe epilepsy is the paroxysmal pattern, as described by Szondi but unknown in American clinical circles.

The relationship between epilepsy and the NDE has been discussed by other investigators, whose work should be examined because they all make differing philosophical assumptions. First, the neurologist Michael Persinger claims that temporal lobe epilepsy and NDEs are variants of a general continuum of psychic seizures. The temporal lobe region comprises projection, visual imagery, hearing, vestibular movements, and sensations of balance, all of which are found in epilepsy and NDEs. Even Moody connects projections to migraines and epilepsy (1988, 124). Persinger cites the following NDE case:

> Suddenly I felt myself being lifted up, like the movement in an elevator. I felt like I was moving down a long corridor—I could see my body slowly moving away from "me." I was spinning around and around in the soft darkness. Then I stopped, it was like floating. At first I felt terror, then I heard a voice and all the fear left. The voice said, "Go back; it's not your time," and *I knew* it was God, I did not want to return; the feeling of infinite peace was all around me and I hated to return to the pain of my life (Persinger 1987, 26-27).

Persinger points out that the sensations of "being lifted up," "floating," "moving," "hearing a voice," and "infinite peace," belong to the temporal lobe seizure syndrome. Absent from the example are the light and meeting deceased relatives, neither of which can be fully explained neurologically. Persinger interprets the NDE as depersonalization caused by instability in the temporal lobe. As argued in section two, this concept does not fully account for the rich feelings and perceptions of the NDE. Persinger's use of the notion depersonalization betrays his philosophical commitment to an epiphenomenal monism, which affirms the primacy of physical reality, derivative status of mind, and the brain as a closed system.

Second, Morse grounds his study in a philosophical dualism, when he posits a soul independent of brain tissues but disclosed through the genetically coded neural circuits (1990, 108). He draws upon the work of Wilder Penfield, who electrically stimulated his patients' right temporal lobe, in the "Sylvian fissure," producing out-of-body states, music, life review, deceased persons, and presence of God. Morse does not assign exclusive priority to the right temporal lobe reactions but to a nonmaterial soul, capable of surviving biological death. However, it is not clear how the independent soul relates to the effects of the electrical stimulation of the brain, which Morse cites in Penfield's work.

Likewise, Michael Sabom appeals to Penfield's work and also frames the NDE in a dualism. Sabom summarizes the characteristics of temporal lobe epilepsy, as established by Penfield: (1) sensory illusions;

(2) feelings of fear, sadness, or loneliness; (3) visual and auditory hallucinations; and (4) forced thinking or crowding of random ideas (1982, 173-174). Assuming these to be definitive of epilepsy, Sabom contrasts them with NDE traits: (1) undistorted perception of the environment; (2) pervasive calm, peace, and joy; (3) absence of taste and smell; (4) life review, comprising a succession of several meaningful elements instead of a single, random event; and (5) absence of forced thinking (174). Sabom concludes that the NDE is not identical to epilepsy, but it involves a psychic mechanism that separates from the body and exists independently of the brain.

Sabom illustrates the contrast between epilepsy and the NDE with two cases. The first involves a "severe infectious illness and grand mal seizure at age fifteen," as recalled by a 73 year old woman:

> Then I became separated and I was sitting way up there looking
> at myself convulsing and my mother and my maid screaming and
> yelling because they thought I was dead. I felt so sorry for them
> and for my body.... Just deep, deep *sadness*. I can still feel the
> sadness. But I felt I was free up there and there was no reason
> for suffering. I had no pain and was completely free (20).

This case clearly contradicts the claim, cited above, that epilepsy has visual hallucinations and distorted thought. The sadness derives from a clear perception of the reactions of the mother and maid, but it is overcome by painlessness and freedom. As with the Dostoevsky aura the conquest of suffering is predominate, so that any conceptual distinction between epilepsy and the NDE collapses.

Secondly, Sabom describes "a grand mal seizure associated with severe toxemia of pregnancy" in a 20 year old woman:

> I knew something was going to happen...and then I went
> unconscious...and I was looking down and could see myself
> going into convulsions, and I was starting to fall out of bed, and
> the girl in the next bed screaming for the nurses.... The nurse
> caught me and put me back and by then there were two other
> nurses there and one came back almost immediately with a
> tongue depressor on my tongue. And they got the sides up on
> the bed and they called the doctor.... It was a feeling of height,
> great distance, a light feeling *like being up in a balcony* looking

down and watching all this and feeling very detached as though
I was watching someone else, like you might watch a movie....
It was a very calm, relaxed feeling, a feeling of well-being if
anything...(29-30).

This case also contradicts Sabom's claim of sensory distortion and fear
in the epileptic seizure. It clearly illustrates the paroxysmal symbolic
motif of height, as well as the stripping away of the body in projective-
participatory being, and the sense of peace in the Dostoevsky aura.

Although Sabom intends to separate NDEs and epilepsy sharply, his
own cases do not support the distinction. The characteristics of epilepsy,
cited by Sabom may be attributed to complex partial seizures, but they
do not correspond to the profound knowledge of epilepsy achieved by the
asylum doctors. Nowhere is the Dostoevsky aura considered in the
discussion of epilepsy. Dostoevsky discovered that the sublime ecstasy
of the aura made distinctions of normal and abnormal irrelevant. Yet he
also discovered the fundamental polarity of epilepsy, joy balanced by
mystic terror, light by darkness, peace by guilt and the dread of
punishment. Dostoevsky knew that mystic terror was the condition to
behold the light, because the goal of the seizure was to manifest
restitution.

It is not my intent to identify epilepsy and the NDE but to derive
them from the paroxysmal pattern, including its polarity of Cain and
Abel tendencies. Grounding these phenomena in the paroxysmal pattern
shows that they are governed by the basic need for atonement in the face
of death. Appealing to the paroxysmal pattern illumines the fact that
negative NDEs fail to achieve restitution, a factor inhibiting participation
in fundamental, transcendent reality.

Monism and dualism are simply inadequate explanations for the
radiant shock of death-related events. Monism presumes the primacy of
physical objective reality, and dualism uncritically retains a dogmatic
conception of death as a separation of soul and body. Despite the aid of
medical technology, investigators employ questionable philosophical
assumptions uncritically. Uncritical thought is further characterized by
the absence of historical scholarship in the NDE literature. When
viewed historically, it becomes apparent that the insights of Albert Heim
in the nineteenth century remain fundamental and still unintegrated in
current discussions.

VIII. MIND AS ACT

In the remainder of this chapter I sketch a theory of the NDE with reference to the foregoing clinical and metaphysical issues. My proposed theory also embraces the dreams and visions of death and grief. A general theory of these phenomena should abandon a view of reality as exhaustively physical, objective, sequential, and locomotive. Such a theory should also give up the attempt to locate mind as an entity, capable of separating from the bodily brain. The conception of mind as entity carries on the older notion of soul as entity as well.

I propose to conceive of mind as act. The principal reason is to explain the primary datum of shock events, namely, acceleration of thought. The classical theory of mind as act was formulated by Susanne Langer, who assumed with Alfred North Whitehead that events are the basic constituents of nature. Within every domain of the universe the act informs all movements and elements. The act is an indivisible whole, consisting of an initial moment, acceleration, consummation, and closing phase (Langer 1967, 291). The potential for the act is the impulse, which is a tendency toward completion. Acts are not isolated events but moments in a series, which unfold in flow patterns characterized by regularity and probability. Acts relate with one another in diverse patterns of interacting. Interacting patterns exhibit contraries and alternates, which appear in rhythms. The various regions of the universe have specific forms of rhythmic interacting. When conceived as a whole, the universe appears to be a vast ocean of wave-like patterns of ebb and flow, undulating forces of energy and mass.

Human life is distinguished by the advanced evolution of feeling, which provides for the specialization of thought through form and imagination. Mind as act comprises feeling and imaginal form. Just as the act rises to a consummation before ending, so, in the same way, feelings need to be completed in imaginal forms (Langer 1972, 285). In this way acts of thought may be felt as well as remembered.

The philosophy of mind as act accounts for current neurobiological models. Contemporary neurology identifies the neuron as the discrete functional unit of the brain. The neuron is a cell with an electrical element and membrane boundary, functioning as an action potential that produces phases of excitation and inhibition. Altogether, the brain comprises billions of individual neurons, each of which releases its own energy in pulsating rhythms of coming into being and passing away.

Consciousness is the wave-like pattern that emerges in the instantaneous firings of the billions of neurons. The flow of consciousness includes the rhythm of neural excitation and inhibition. The phase of excitation generates feeling and form according to the paroxysmal pattern, as it applies both to dreams and to epileptic seizures.

Langer's definition of the act conforms precisely to Szondi's conception of paroxysmality. The paroxysmal excitation of the brain coincides with acceleration of thought amid shock events. Since the concept of act informs thought fundamentally, then the entitative notions of brain and mind are derivative. To conceptualize events in terms of brain and mind as entities puts the issues on a secondary level of reflection. Consequently, monism and dualism are equally derivative and beside the point. Because acting is relating and relating is rhythmic, there is no need to distinguish the physical from the psychological aspects of the brain. Functions in the brain are themselves derivative from the wave-like rhythms of feeling and form.

In the shock of mortal danger the paroxysmal excitatory function of the brain dominates while sensory-muscular systems and pain stimuli are inhibited. The startle network is the starter, igniting thought to accelerate. The shock accelerates thought to such an intensity that the order of space and time, extension and succession recedes. The dynamics of thought acceleration have been suggested in a letter by Carl Jung:

> It might be that the psyche should be understood as *unextended intensity* and not as a body moving with time. One might assume the psyche gradually arising from minute extensity to infinite intensity, transcending for instance the velocity of light and thus irrealizing the body.... (1975, 45)

Here Jung understands the brain as a transformer station, in which the intensity of mind turns into perceptible frequencies or extensions. This is a helpful idea, and I would add that the ego phases, such as projection and introjection are also grounded in the frequencies.

My explanation of thought-acceleration correlates with Albert Einstein's theory of relativity. When systems are accelerated from rest, they cannot be accelerated beyond the speed of light. This postulate excludes those systems, in which particles do not accelerate but move at the speed of light as soon as they exist, such as neutrinos and photons.

Einstein's postulate does not exclude tachyons or supraluminal particles, even though they may not be confirmed experimentally. Nevertheless, a rod accelerating up to the speed of light would disappear, and a clock, moving at the same velocity, would become slower and eventually stop when reaching the speed of light.

By analogy, when thought accelerates to a higher-level intensity, it becomes luminous, approaching the speed of light, as it were. Since the speed of light is not an absolute limit, the possibility of supraluminous intensity remains open for radiant forms of dream, vision, and telepathy. As thought accelerates, simultaneously, spatial extension vanishes, and temporal succession slows down to a point. The body is no longer felt, because its form has been transcended; thus, the light that radiates in the NDE is the accelerated intensity of thought itself.

Through the acceleration of thought, the radiant shock of death reveals fundamental reality. In current cosmology the universe is understood as a flowing, indivisible whole of energy, which may be symbolized by a vast ocean (Bohm 1980, 210). The same symbol appears in the thought of Frederic Myers, William James, and Carl Jung. All life arises from the cosmic sea of energy. Local space-time regions shape the order of daily life, but they are derivative and dissolve into the oceanic background of energy at death. Location is a limited and abstract representation of a region but not fundamental. When humans confront the threat of death, their thought processes accelerate to luminous intensities and change into their essential and unextended beings. Having ignited the paroxysmal pattern, the shock of death culminates the primal drive for participation in social and metaphysical reality.

IX. ARCHETYPAL PARTICIPATION

When Raymond Moody published his original NDE case studies, he suggested parallels between them and the history of religions, particularly the Bible, Tibetan Book of the Dead, and the visions of Emanuel Swedenborg (1975, 111-128). These citations are not stated on the basis of critical scholarship, but they do suggest the cross-cultural experience of the light. The cumulative research findings, conducted since Moody's initial publication, also confirm the primacy of light in the NDE.

Appropriately, Moody's suggestions stimulated scholars to find historical parallels to the NDE. One of the most definitive works is

Carol Zaleski's study, claiming that the NDE is the current version of the classical otherworld journey (1987). She argues that the otherworld journey of the ancient Shaman is the prototype and that it is associated with initiatory death and rebirth rituals. She illustrates her argument with the classical Christian otherworld journey, which comprises the following stages: (1) exit from the body; (2) encounter with a spiritual guide or gate keeper; (3) travel to heaven, purgatory, or hell; (4) confronting obstacles (e.g. fire, mountains), test bridge, and weighing of deeds; (5) followed by re-entry, with a command to return, personal transformation, and narrative recollection of the event (45-77). She interprets the otherworld journey as a form of imagination, intended to maintain a mythic model of the cosmos and to offer guidance to people during cultural crises (192-204).

By comparing the Moody type NDE to the classical Christian otherworld journey, Zaleski demonstrates convincingly that diverse symbols shape the phenomena in different cultural periods. For example, the older type has the two deaths motif, according to which an easy exit from the body signifies a saintly character, but agony denotes a sinner. The current version has only a pleasant exit. The older form features a hierarchy of being, reflecting the stratification of Medieval society. In the current model everyone is equal. Whereas in the older type, persons receive commands; in the newer one people are given choices whether to live or to die.

While Zaleski's book deals mainly with Western Christian civilization, an earlier study grounded the NDE in four archetypes of the history of religions: (1) One enters an out-of-body state and becomes a spiritual body, inaudible, invisible, and nonmaterial. In this essential being one floats or hovers over the corpse. (2) One meets deceased relatives or friends. (3) The meeting coincides with the encounter of a border, limit, or dividing line toward which one crosses over the water by means of a boat, bridge, or rainbow. (4) One beholds the light (Holck 1978-1979).

In my view, the Holck study rather than the Zaleski comes first in the order of historical priorities. The Holck paper identifies the cross-over pattern, which, as archeology demonstrates, is an archaic archetype derived from the perceived cycle of the sun. In the primeval imagination the sun moved across the sky to the Western horizon before descending below the earth to begin the otherworld journey (Lauf 1980, 89-91). Journey as descent preceded that of ascent, which informs the Zaleski and Moody types. The otherworld journey as an ascent informed ancient Greco-Roman culture, whereas that of descent occurred in the ancient Near East.

The four primordial archetypes, identified by the Holck study, reflect the basic paroxysmal shock symbols. The motif of crossing over to a border or floating through a tunnel represents the archetype of water. Radiant light is an expression of fire. The darkness of the tunnel or void signifies an epileptiform loss of consciousness in the sense of "blacking out." The transition from darkness to light is also epileptiform, and it signifies a shift from an unconscious to a transpersonal state. The Dostoevsky aura is the standard.

Meeting deceased relatives and friends is not so much archetypal as genotropic and familial. Friends are gene relatives who, along with blood relatives, occupy the familial unconscious. In the Moody type of NDE the relatives are bathed in light, which means that the ancestors dwell in the supraluminous threshold of accelerated thought forms. The ancestors attain in death an unextended psychic intensity, the forms of which are preserved in the generations of the family. These ancestral forms enter the dreams and visions of descendants, in accord with the biological principle that organisms strive to perpetuate their genes in subsequent generations.

It is well-known that Moody personalizes the Being of Light and defines it theologically as God, Christ, or angel (1975, 59). Naming the Being of Light as divine is intended to support his contention of parallels between the Bible and the NDE (112-113). However, designating the Being of Light as God is a theological judgment that surpasses the boundaries of clinical methodology. It is questionable with respect to the biblical tradition, which assigns priority to darkness, an issue to be explored further in chapter seven.

In contrast to Moody's opinion, I suggest that the Being of Light manifests the pontifical ego or participatory selfhood. Since the light emanates from the tunnel, which derives from the archaic cross-over pattern, then the most precise historical parallel would be the Persian Chinvat Bridge, on which the deceased discovers his or her destiny as a radiant being of light (*Daena*). The Being of Light, discovered on the bridge or its equivalents, is one's own primal form, projected as a radiant intensity, culminating the acceleration of thought, and creating participation in fundamental metaphysical reality.

To illustrate the relation between the bridge and the light, a case reported by a nurse and cardiologist is considered. The nurse was a former student of mine who took care of an 81 year old male. He sustained an extensive myocardial infarction and was admitted to a coronary care unit. While there, he suffered two nonfatal cardiac arrests, the first lasting 32 seconds and the second 23. In each instance he left his body with the knowledge of his own death and travelled on a beam of light:

> Ahead of him, the beam stretched to infinity, at what appeared to be a forty-five degree angle and was aimed upward. On each side of the beam was a dark abyss. As he moved with the beam of light, he described sensing the most beautiful colors imaginable which were present in the beam of light, but were unlike colors on earth.
>
> Accompanying the light was an "eerie" sound, and he described the sound as a whistling sound, as if it were possible to hear the speed of light. He stated that he did not encounter any people and did not hear any voices, only this eerie, rushing sound.

For this man, who "died" twice, the light unfolded as a rainbow bridge, spanning a dark unconscious abyss. The uncanny sound echoed the shock of his own psyche accelerating into luminous archetypal form. In two NDEs he became a radiant being, with exalted participatory power, beyond unfathomable waters of the cosmic sea.

CHAPTER SEVEN:
DEATH, MOURNING, AND REJOICING

I. LAND OF NO RETURN

Beginning with this chapter our study of death as a shock event turns to the theological sources, specifically, to the Bible. Generally, the ancient Hebrews conceived of death as a dissolution of the whole human being, a draining of its vitality, and a scattering of its power (Silberman 1969, 19-20). Life was conceived as a whole, and its vital power extended from the individual to the community, offspring, and property. Death was a breaking of this extensive continuum but not an extinction. Death was not so much a separation event but a variety of states of powerlessness or weakness. If the body were struck down by a traumatic force, some vitality could persist in scattered parts of the whole. If death were by murder, then the vital fragments would evoke the need for retribution.

Before the fall of Samaria, in 722-721 B.C.E. the Hebrews considered death to be the natural end of the life span, under the following conditions: (1) the deceased had lived a normal span of time (Gen. 6:3, 120 years; Ps. 90:10, 70 years); (2) had left behind children for mourning and remembrance; and (3) had been buried in a grave to prevent vengeance by the corpse and disruption of the order of the world (Jacob 1962, 802). Normally, burial took place in a rock-cut, chamber tomb, belonging to the family of the deceased.

Abraham represented this natural type of death; he lived 175 years and was "buried in a good old age" (Gen. 15:15; 25:7), as did Job, who died "old and full of days" (Jb. 42:17). The phrase "gathered to your kin" also designated a natural death, and it referred to national leaders like Moses and Aaron (Deut. 32:50). The phrase "to sleep with one's ancestors" indicated the natural death of kings, primarily in the books of Kings (I Kgs. 14:20; 15:24; 22:40, 50) and Chronicles (II Chron. 9:31; 12:16; 16:13; 27:9). Likewise, the phrases "to lie down in death" and "lying in the grave" meant a natural death. That these phrases are indirect verbal statements implies the Hebrew belief that dying was involuntary.

The Hebrews imagined the dead occupying a region below the earth called Sheol, an underground pit, where all the individual graves intersected. The idea of Sheol was inferred from burial practice, and it coincided with the earliest conception of a "beyond" in the Old Testament (Tromp 1969, 23). Sheol could be regarded as an unconscious realm that erupts into life, as long as this idea were not hypostatized as "the Unconscious." In any case, Sheol would conform to the notion of the familial unconscious, in as much as burial meant joining the ancestors.

The Hebrews thought of death in relation to their neighbors, particularly the Canaanites, who conceived of the underworld as a city, whose name *Hmry* meant "pit" or "abyss" in Ugaritic and Hebrew cognates (Astour 1980, 229). The underground city was ruled by Mot, the Canaanite god of death and a voracious monster with large dangerous jaws that extend from the earth to the heavens and the stars. Mot has lips and tongue, throat, stomach and limbs; he is a personal, demonic being who rises up from the underground to swallow the living violently. Thus, Canaanite mythology projects the image of death as killing and eating.

Although Sheol resembled *Hmry*, the Hebrews could not assimilate entirely the Canaanite mythology of death. The Hebrews' settlement in Palestine, where they met the Canaanites, was governed by the Mosaic prohibition of other gods (Ex. 20:3-4). Since no other gods were permissible in Israel, the Hebrews "broke" the mythology of death but retained some of its shock-images. Various Canaanite images were grafted onto the notion of Sheol enabling the people to face realistically the eruptive horror of death.

Some of the richest images of Sheol are found in the Psalms and the book of Job. Sheol lies in "the depths of the earth," which is balanced by "the heights of the mountains" (Ps. 95:4). Since the roots of the mountains penetrate the earth, they shake with God's anger: "The foundations also of the mountains trembled and quaked, because he was angry. Smoke went up from his nostrils, and devouring fire from his mouth; glowing coals flamed forth from him" (Ps. 18:76-78). Sheol contains many pits, into which the wicked fall, when hit by burning coals (Ps. 140:10).

To die is to go "down into the depths" (Ps. 107:26a). The notion of depth emphasizes the unbridgeable gulf between the living and the dead. Sinking into the depths also accounts for any weakness, suffering, sickness, or distress. Weakness is like falling, being dragged down to low or distant places. These images of "going down" and "falling" are paroxysmal conceptions of death as a shock-event.

Many of the images of death entail the shock symbol of the earth. Job says of the dead: "Hide them all in the dust together, bind their faces in the world below" (40:13). Hiding faces means to suppress their personalities. Similarly, Isaiah proclaims: "Then deep from the earth you shall speak, from low in the dust your words shall come; your voice shall come from the ground like the voice of a ghost, and your speech shall whisper out of the dust" (29:4).

Generally, the Old Testament distinguishes between earth, ground, and dust. In the Creation Narrative dust signifies transitoriness; for after Adam eats the fruit of the Tree of Knowledge, God declares: "You are dust and to dust you shall return" (Gen. 3:19b). Earth lies beneath the "dust of the ground" (*Adamah*), from which the man (Adam) has been created (Gen. 2:7a). Terms for the ground and man are related, the former feminine and the latter masculine. The divine breath or spirit flows from the man into the ground and binds them into a unity.

The bond is broken, however, when Cain murders his brother Abel. The ground "opened its mouth to receive your brother's blood from your hand" (Gen. 4:11). The blood flows out of the corpse into the ground, rupturing the primal bond and poisoning the earth. The image of the ground swallowing Abel's blood reflects the Canaanite myth of the devouring jaws of Mot. Thereafter, death remains the "Hungry One" of the desert. Job explains that their "strength is consumed by hunger, and calamity is ready for their stumbling. By disease their skin is consumed, the firstborn of Death consumes their limbs" (18:12-13). Anyone who is so consumed becomes a mythic son of Mot.

The Creation Narrative also employs the shock symbol of water, as it relates to Sheol. "In the beginning when God created the heavens and the earth, the earth was a formless void and darkness covered the face of the deep, while a wind from God swept over the face of the waters"

(Gen. 1:1-2). Here the primeval ocean (*Tehom*) is supported by the massive earth yet encircles it; and its waves surge with elemental force, always ready to threaten chaos (Tromp 1969, 44, 59, 61). The primeval ocean has a subterranean connection with Sheol: "For the waves of death encompassed me, the torrents of perdition assailed me; the cords of Sheol entangled me, the snares of death confronted me" (II Sam. 22:5-6).

Still other passages combine elements of earth and water to imagine the terror of Sheol. The desolate pit contains watery sands, quicksand, and a "miry bog" (Ps. 40:2). The pit is like a muddy cistern (Jer. 38:6). Sinking into the muddy waters conceals the dead from the face of God (Ps. 143:7) and traps them behind prison bars (Jon. 2:6). The miry bog and muddy waters destroy all hope; for they lie in the deepest place, an unfathomable abyss, falling into which brings only ruin and destruction.

The eruptive force of the abyss is well expressed in Psalm 124, where death as the savage enemy would "swallow us up alive" (v. 3), "flood would have swept us away" (v. 4), "given us as prey to their teeth" (v. 6), and "the snare of the fowlers" (v. 7). Hidden in the muddy waters, miry bog, or desolate pit, death lurks ever ready to seize, strike, and slay.

Behind the oldest texts, an archaic cosmology links Sheol with the desert, the ocean, and the night as the zones of death (Pedersen 1926, 458-459). The desert is the place of death due to the loss of fertility in the ground, after the murder of Abel, and it is indistinguishable from the wilderness: "my soul thirsts for you; my flesh faints for you, as in a dry and weary land where there is no water" (Ps. 63:1b). However, the Old Testament does not equate death with the desert exclusively, because Sheol is mainly a watery place with channels to the primeval ocean.

Several passages in Job view Sheol as night or darkness: "before I go, never to return, to the land of gloom and deep darkness, the land of gloom and chaos, where light is like darkness" (10:21-22); "they are thrust from light into darkness and driven out of the world" (18:18); "they despair of returning from darkness" (15:22); and he "has set darkness upon my paths" (19:8b).

Sheol has two mountains standing at the border, where a river flows along a border. To die is to cross the river. Job declares the river to be a place of judgment: "that he may turn them aside from their deeds, and keep them from pride, to spare their souls from the Pit, their lives from traversing the River" (33:17-18). Since the river is absent in Canaanite mythology, Job's description reflects the influence of Mesopotamian thought. In Mesopotamian mythology the river is called *Hubur*. It flows at the edge of the earth, at the Western horizon, which is reached after crossing a vast, barren desert. The water of *Hubur* encircles the earth and separates this world from the dark shores of the beyond. Those shores are so distant, so poorly discerned, that one does not know whether they be above or below the primeval ocean (Bottero 1980, 31-32).

In Mesopotamian mythology the dead cross the river *Hubur* and, once going beyond the dismal banks of water, they enter the land of no return. Beyond the frontier the dead find an immense, muddy, obscure cavern, where they dwell in darkness, immobility, and silence. The context is essentially the same in the Old Testament wherein, upon burial, the dead cross the river, which is like an underground tunnel, and are forgotten. For "there is no work or thought or knowledge or wisdom in Sheol, to which you are going" (Eccles. 9:10). God's face is hidden from those in the land of forgetfulness (Ps. 88:12, 14). The dead have neither joy nor possessions (Jb. 15:29). The dead dwell in the land of no return: "Can I bring him back again? I shall go to him, but he will not return to me" (II Sam. 12:23).

II. DESCENT TO SHEOL AND MOURNING

The various images of Sheol in the Old Testament coalesce into the paroxysmal symbolic motif of descent. In the Bible and the ancient Near East the image of descent corresponded to prescribed rituals of mourning. Thus, Sheol refers not only to the underground pit but also to grief. The mythic image projects what the community acts out ritually.

The same ritual context appears in Canaanite mythology, when Mot slays his brother Baal, the god of fertility. El, the Supreme god and father of Baal and Mot, begins to grieve:

Then El the kind, the compassionate:
descends from the throne and sits on the footstool,
    from the footstool and [descends and] sits upon the
            ground.
He strews stalks of mourning on his head,

the dust in which he wallows on his pate.
His clothing he tears, down to the loin cloth,
   his skin he bruises with a rock by pounding,
   with a razor he cuts his beard and whiskers,
He rakes his upper arms,
   he plows his breast like a garden,
   like a valley he rakes his chest.
He raises his voice and shouts:
"Baal is dead: What will happen to the people?
   Dogon's son: What will happen to the masses?
I am descending to the underworld, after Baal"
(Anderson 1991, 60-63).

Anat, the sister and consort of Baal, grieves as well, and she descends to the underworld, going by way of the edge of the desert at the Western horizon and accompanied by Shapshu, the sun-goddess. Anat seizes and slays Mot, thereby freeing Baal and restoring him to the world of the living. The restoration of Baal requires the cessation of mourning and the return to social life, as announced by El:

In a dream of El the Kind, the compassionate,
   in a vision of the Creator of all,
the heavens rained down oil
   the wadis ran with honey
El the kind, the compassionate was glad:
   he put his feet on a stool,
he opened his mouth and laughed;
   he raised his voice and shouted;
"I now take my seat and rest,
   my soul rests within me,
because Baal the conqueror lives,
   the Prince, the lord of the earth is alive!"
(Anderson 1991, 67)

Mourning is also explored in the Mesopotamian Epic of Gilgamesh. Gilgamesh, King of Uruk and two-thirds divine, suffers the death of his friend Enkidu, who had learned of his impending death through a precognitive dream (Tab. 7; Col. 4):

He seized me and led me down to the house of darkness...
The house where one who goes in never comes out again,
The road that, if one takes it, one never comes back,
The house that, if one lives there, one never sees light,
The place where they live on dust, their food is mud
(Gardner and Maier, 1984, 178).

When Enkidu dies after his dream, Gilgamesh is devastated and realizes that he too will die one day (Tab. 9; Col. 1):

Gilgamesh for his friend Enkidu bitterly cried. He roamed the hills. "Me! Will I too not die like Enkidu? Sorrow has come into my belly. I fear death; I roam over the hills. I will seize the road...." (Gardner and Maier 1984, 196)

This passage portrays Gilgamesh crossing the Steppe, which is the same as descending into the underworld (Bottero 1980, 32). The crossing implies a state of shock and panic; for Gilgamesh cries, pulls out his hair, takes off his clothing, puts on lions' skins, and refuses to eat food. Such actions mean that Gilgamesh has regressed to a primal state of nature, which Enkidu originally represented (Tigay 1982, 202-203). Enkidu had walked the Steppe with wild animals, was hairy, ate grass, and did not like human food. His friendship with Gilgamesh had been a part of his humanization. Clinically, the grieving of Gilgamesh reveals a mania and contact-seeking for the lost "object" and for immortality, as a conquest of death.

However, Gilgamesh encounters Siduri, the bar-maid, and he explains to her (Tab. 10; Col. 2):

Enkidu whom I love dearly underwent with me all hardships. The fate of mankind overtook him. Six days and seven nights I wept over him until a worm fell out of his nose. Then I was afraid. In fear of death I roam the wilderness (Gardner and Maier 1984, 212).

This passage confirms a ritually prescribed period of seven days of mourning and indicates that Gilgamesh grieves beyond that limit. He who has delayed burial, kept searching for the deceased, and wandered the Steppe has identified with the dead and exhibited acute chronic grief.

Gilgamesh's lament for Enkidu resounds throughout the underworld in hope that the deceased would return within the seven day period (Müller 1978, 243).

In reply, Siduri explains to Gilgamesh that no mortal can cross the sea and the wilderness to immortality; only Shamash, the sun-god, can do that. She then counsels Gilgamesh to give up looking for immortality:

> As for you, Gilgamesh, let your belly be full,
> Make merry day and night.
> Of each day make a feast of rejoicing,
> Day and night dance and play!
> Let your garments be sparkling fresh,
> Your head be washed; bathe in water.
> Pay heed to a little one that holds on to your hand.
> Let a spouse delight in your bosom.
> For this is the task of [woman] (Tigay 1982, 168).

Siduri's speech is found in the Old Babylonian version and not in the later text. She insists that he should cease grieving and take up the rituals of rejoicing which are basic to civilized life.

Both Canaanite and Gilgamesh stories illustrate the fact that the mythic imagery of death correlates with a specific ritual of mourning set in opposition to rituals of life. Behavior common to the living is vigorously avoided so as not to antagonize the dead. The mythic ritual of mourning has been compared to the anthropological rite of passage: (1) death as separation, laying out of the corpse, and burial; (2) transitional phase consisting of grieving for seven days and nights; and (3) reincorporation of the bereaved into society, including the completion of grieving (Anderson 1991, 77). This correlation is helpful only in the sense that the rite of passage pertains to normal grief. Gilgamesh goes beyond that limit with chronic grief.

The Canaanite and Gilgamesh ritual settings were consistent with those in the Old Testament. A seven day and night period of mourning was common in ancient Israel (I Sam. 31:13). However, Deuteronomy extended the seven day period to one of thirty days (34:8), a phase practiced in modern Jewish rituals. In ancient Israel when death was announced, survivors tore their garments and put on rough clothing (II Sam. 1:11; 3:3; II Kgs. 6:30). They took off their shoes and headdress, shaved their hair (Isa. 15:2; II Sam. 10:4; Jer. 41:5), cut their bodies, and sprinkled their heads and faces with dirt (Neh. 9:1). Mourners neither washed nor groomed themselves but wore sackcloth and fasted (Ps. 35:13).

The bereaved could address the deceased with a kinship metaphor, such as, "Alas, my brother" (I Kgs. 13:30) or with a confession of love, as with "greatly beloved" (II Sam. 1:26). The lament for the deceased could include a recitation of virtues, such as "swifter than eagles...stronger than lions" (II Sam. 1:23b). Metaphors of a lamentation stress a sharp difference between what was and what is now: "How the mighty have fallen" (II Sam. 1:19, 25, 27). The entire community is invited to mourn, so as to share the grief: "O daughter of Israel, weep...." (II Sam. 1:24a)

The Old Testament narrates specific symptoms of grief. The bereaved is "bowed down," suffers "burning loins, "groans, feels crushed, sighs" (Ps. 38:6-10). One feels that "joy is gone, grief is upon me, my heart is sick" (Jer. 8:18). While grieving for several days, one falls down to the ground (II Sam. 14:2, 4). The falling would in the European Middle Ages be interpreted as a sign of epilepsy in grief (Temkin 1971, 112).

The Old Testament also reports situations in which mourning exceeds the seven day limit and continues indefinitely. For example, when Jacob discovers his son Joseph missing and his robe torn into pieces:

> Then Jacob tore his garments, and put sackcloth on his loins, and mourned for his son many days. All his sons and all his daughters sought to comfort him; but he refused to be comforted, and said, "no, I shall go down to Sheol to my son, mourning" (Gen. 37:34-35).

Jacob's descent into Sheol is the same as Gilgamesh wandering across the wilderness. Both episodes demonstrate acute chronic grief.

The Old Testament agrees with the Gilgamesh epic that the state of morbid or chronic grief is separated from civilization and from God. The Psalmist complains that he cannot praise God in Sheol: "I am weary with my moaning; every night I flood my bed with tears; I drench my couch with my weeping" (Ps. 6:6). Still the Psalmist pleads for deliverance:

With your faithful help rescue me from sinking in the mire; let me be delivered from my enemies and from the deep waters. Do not let the flood sweep over me, or the deep swallow me up, or the Pit close its mouth over me (Ps. 69:13b-15).

Deliverance from Sheol is an occasion for rejoicing (Ps. 16:9-11). The Psalmist expresses a fixed, ritual form of lamentation, followed by praise. The intent of the lament is to remove suffering and that of praise is to make an offering and anticipate the future (Kugel 1986, 123). For example,

...from the depths of the earth you will bring me up again. You will increase my honor, and comfort me once again.
I will praise you with the harp for your faithfulness, O my God; I will sing praises to you with the lyre, O Holy One of Israel (Ps. 71:20b-22).

Psalm 107 specifies thanksgiving as well as praise for deliverance from the zones of Sheol, for those who "wander in desert wastes" (v. 4a), "prisoners in misery and in irons" (v. 10b), and for those who "went down to the sea in ships, doing business on the mighty waters" (v. 23). Although lamentation and praise are oriented toward different spheres, the urgency and intensity of each are the same (Müller 1978, 239).

Nevertheless, the Old Testament maintains a polar dichotomy of praise and lamentation. Whereas mourners grieve for seven days (Gen. 50:10), the assembly keeps a festival for seven days with gladness (II Chron. 30: 23; Neh. 12:27). Festivals of praise include eating and drinking, sexual relationships, anointing with oil, and wearing festal clothing, all of which are prohibited to mourners. The bereaved are excluded from public rituals of praise and may rejoice only in the future, when grief ceases (Ps. 137). Eating, drinking, and anointing with oil signify the end of mourning as well as deliverance from death (Isa. 35:10). Rejoicing after deliverance is the meaning of being comforted (Ps. 86:17; Ps. 71:20-21).

The reason for the dichotomy of rejoicing and grieving has to do with the status of the will. In the Old Testament the term for joy (*Simha*) is interchangeable with that for will (Muffs 1975, 11). For example, in Hebrew law a contract becomes valid only when both parties smile. A radiant face shows willingness and no regret. Here is the origin of projection, namely, the Hebrew belief that the face represents one's inner thoughts. Should one frown or be sad, a contract becomes void, because sadness indicates unwillingness. Thus, the bereaved are excluded from rituals of rejoicing, because they suffer an impairment of the will. Mourning ends, when the bereaved are willing and able "to rejoice in the Lord."

III. CROSS-OVER SYMBOLS AND THE TEMPLE

In ancient Mesopotamia Shamash, the sun-god, had the power to travel the desert to the Western horizon, descend to the underworld, go through the tunnel, and reappear the next morning at the Eastern horizon. For the living, Shamash is known as the helper and protector of travellers:

Illuminator, dispeller of darkness of the *vault* of the heavens, who sets aglow the beard of light, the corn field, the life of the lord. Regularly and without cease you traverse the heavens. Every day you pass over the broad earth. The flood of the sea, the mountains, the earth, the heavens (Lambert 1960, 127).

The sun deity is clearly distinguished from the hero. In Mesopotamia Gilgamesh cannot cross the "waters of death," even with the aid of Shamash. In Canaanite mythology Shapshu accompanies Anat into the underworld in search of the slain Baal. These patterns prove that the hero myth cannot be identified with the cross-over pattern of the sun, as in the case in Jungian psychology. Further, ancient Near Eastern myth designates the Western horizon as the realm of death, in accord with the primeval crossing of the sun and with the desert journey as a form of death. However, the ancient Near East differs from British and Scandinavian symbolism in one basic respect. By means of projection the underworld is imagined as a counterpart to the sun's crossing and as an underground tunnel, through which the sun deity returns (Healey 1980). British and Scandinavian symbolism did not clearly specify an underworld journey.

Further, within Mesopotamia the sun god had the power of necromancy, which is the ability to derive knowledge from the dead. The dead came as apparitions, dream-forms, or hauntings in a ceaseless procession, thus contradicting the idea of death as "the land of no return." The apparent cause of such manifestations was the absence of burial (Bottero 1980, 40-41). The rituals focused on the skull; that is, the sun deity would speak through a skull of the deceased, who in turn, would return through it. Some rituals were used to prevent the apparitions of the dead from occurring. One text describes the skull being kissed or licked to prevent the grinding of teeth during sleep (Finkel 1983-1984, 14). This suggests that the dead returned to the living through epileptic seizures.

Although necromancy took place in Israel, (I Sam. 28) it was forbidden in the normative Mosaic tradition (Deut. 18:11). Whereas in the archaic period of Israel, the dead were thought to occupy Sheol totally alienated from God, the prophets proclaimed that God himself descended into Sheol (I Sam. 2:6; Amos 9:2a). Therefore, necromancy came into conflict with the power of God.

The prophets introduced into Israel a new vision of God as the Divine Warrior, who occupies a throne in the heavenly courtroom, surrounded by members of the divine council (I Kgs. 22:19-23). The prophets proclaimed God as supreme over the elements and over the gods of the ancient Near Eastern mythologies. The power of the Divine Warrior was displayed in the unique biblical form of the cross-over pattern, beginning with the Creation Narrative, in which "a wind from God swept over the face of the waters" (Gen. 1:2b). Thus, the primal act of Creation involved a crossing over the elements of chaos, an act which simultaneously was a release of power over the realm of the dead.

The primeval cross-over of Creation was reenacted in the Exodus, when God commanded Moses and Aaron to perform a blood sacrifice, after which he "will pass through the land of Egypt that night, and I will strike down every firstborn in the land of Egypt...." (Ex. 12:12a) This night of terror allows the Hebrews to escape from bondage in Egypt and cross over the Reed Sea by means of the ebb and flow of the water:

> The Lord drove the sea back by a strong east wind all night, and turned the sea into dry land; and the waters were divided. The Israelites went into the sea on dry ground, the waters forming a wall for them on their right and on their left. The Egyptians pursued, and went into the sea after them....(Ex. 14:21b, 22, 23a)

The Egyptian army became stuck in the mud; i.e. they descended into the miry bog of Sheol. Then Moses stretched out his hand, and the waters returned, drowning the Egyptians (Ex. 14:27-28). The waters that submerged the Egyptians were the same waters over which the Spirit of God crossed at Creation.

The triumph of the Divine Warrior in the Exodus anticipated the Revelation of the Law on Mt. Sinai and, after settling in Canaan, the establishment of the Temple. Solomon constructed the First Temple as a "bridge" between the divine and earth, since it was built according to the heavenly model (Ex. 25-9, 40; 26:30; 27:8). The Psalmist exclaims: "The Lord is in his holy Temple; the Lord's throne is in heaven. His eyes behold, his gaze examines humankind" (11:4).

The Temple liturgy celebrated the enthronement of the Divine Warrior, and it included sacrifices and acts of praise as recalled in the Psalter. Rejoicing in the temple was a public act of avowal, comparable to the royal custom of inscribing words on public monuments (Kugel 1986, 126-127). By rejoicing one created a verbal monument, establishing a participation in the presence of God and standing in opposition to the inscriptions on the walls of tombs. The Temple liturgy also conquered death, and this conquest was signified by the holy water in the courtyard, waters representing the primal sea of chaos, the abyss of Creation (I Kgs. 7:23-26; Ps. 74:12-17).

The prophet Isaiah integrated the presence of the Divine Warrior and the Temple with his vision of the Holy.

> ...I saw the Lord sitting on a throne, high and lofty; and the hem of his robe filled the Temple. Seraphs were in attendance above him...And one called to another and said: "Holy, holy, holy, is the Lord of hosts; the whole earth is full of his glory." The pivots on the thresholds shook at the voices of those who called, and the house filled with smoke. And I said: "Woe is me! I am lost, for I am a man of unclean lips"....(Isa. 6:1b-2a, 3-4)

The prophet's stammering reflects that of Moses before the "Burning Bush" (Ex. 4:10) as a form of stuttering, which is a psychic equivalent of epilepsy (Szondi 1973, 106). Only an angel can cleanse Isaiah's stuttering and allow him to stand in the presence of the holy.

Isaiah formulated an admission liturgy, which featured the divine fire: "Who among us can live with the devouring fire? Who among us can live with everlasting flames?" (Isa. 33:14b). Since the age of the patriarchs, fire had been the divine element in covenant-making (Gen. 15:17-18a; Ex. 3:2; 19:18). Fire emanated from the Spirit of Creation and became an agent of divine revelation: "you make the winds your messengers, fire and flame your ministers" (Ps. 104:4).

Isaiah also formulated a historical eschatology, using Canaanite mythic images and cross-over motifs. He envisaged God's ultimate conquest of death and the cessation of mourning: "he will swallow up death forever. Then the Lord will wipe away the tears from all faces...." (Isa. 25:7b-8a) The end of mourning coincides with the resurrection of the dead: "Your dead shall live, their corpses shall rise. O dwellers in the dust, awake and sing for joy!" (Isa. 26:19a)

The Divine Warrior will defeat the demonic forces of death. "On that day the Lord with his cruel and great and strong sword will punish Leviathan the fleeing serpent, Leviathan the twisting serpent, and he will kill the dragon that is in the sea" (Isa. 27:1). This passage restates the Canaanite myth of Baal, who slays the "Crooked Serpent, the seven-headed beast of the sea" (Gray 1961, 132). In the oracle of Isaiah the serpentine monster is a transpersonal force of death and chaos. It anticipates an impending catastrophe in the history of Israel, namely, the Babylonian Exile (586-538 B.C.E.), when political subjugation by a foreign power prevented the realization of historical eschatology. When the words of the prophets could not be carried out historically, then the vision of the Divine Warrior shifted to a transcendent visionary plane, and apocalyptic eschatology came into being.

IV. DREAMS AND VISIONS OF THE NIGHT

In the Old Testament epochal cross-over events take place at night (e.g. Passover); and the same theme occurs in the New Testament (e.g. the birth of Jesus). Since the night reflects Sheol, cross-over events are full of danger and intrigue. In the history of religions the night is an archetype with three symbolic forms: (1) a time of terror, oppressive silence, or death; (2) a time of oblivion, as in sleep or death; and (3) a time of revelation (Bleeker 1963, 74-76). As a time of revelation, the night is sacred.

Night is primordial; for in the Creation Narrative it comes from the darkness of the abyss (Gen. 1:5). Biblical revelation occurs at night through dreams and visions (I Sam. 3). Between the Revelation of the

Law on Mt. Sinai and the settlement in Canaan, God says he speaks directly to Moses but indirectly to the prophets through dreams and visions (Num. 12:6-8). The same linking of dream and vision is confirmed by the prophet Joel (2:28), who declares: "Your old men shall dream dreams, and your young men shall see visions." The purpose of dreams and visions is explained by Job:

> For God speaks in one way, and in two, though people do not perceive it. In a dream, in a vision of the night, when deep sleep falls on mortals, while they slumber on their beds, then he opens their ears, and terrifies them with warnings, that he may turn them aside from their deeds, and keep them from pride, to spare their souls from the Pit, their lives from traversing the River (33:14-18).

A vision is an experience of an event that is not present and that reveals an immediate understanding, regardless of distance and sense perception (Pedersen 1926, 141). This definition presupposes that life is a whole and that all events are interrelated. Dreams are like visions in the sense that they disclose potentialities for coming occurrences. There is no distinction between dream and action; for dreamwork is expressed in the perfect tense as completed action. The specific dream content may be that of a promise, prediction, or mandate. For example, Jacob is promised offspring in the context of a ladder that "bridges" heaven and earth (Gen. 28:10-16). Dreams of Joseph (Gen. 37:5-11) and Pharaoh (Gen. 41:1-45) predict events symbolically and need to be interpreted. Solomon's dream at Gibeon mandates for him "a wise and discerning mind, riches and honor," if he keeps the statutes and commandments (I Kgs. 3:4-15).

The Bible grants priority to visions and treats dreams critically. The Mosaic tradition governs the interpretation of dreams. If one were to practice divination through dreams, thereby deriving knowledge from other gods, then one would be put to death for treason (Deut. 13:1-5). The standard of dreams is divine truth (Jer. 23:23-28).

As preparation for revelation through dreams and visions, a period of deprivation like mourning was recommended. When waiting for the Sinai Revelation in the desert, the Hebrews cleansed themselves for three days (Ex. 19:10, 15), and Moses fasted forty days and forty nights, even lying prostrate (Deut. 9:9, 18). When Moses ascended the mountain to receive the Revelation, his face was lowered; after receiving it, he descended and his face shone (Ex. 34:28-35). Moses' radiance confirms the Revelation as a gift of joy, an act in which God had no reservations (Muffs 1975, 26-27). The joy is a revelation of God's everlasting willingness.

During the Babylonian Exile, Ezekiel had a great vision of the divine glory and the throne chariot (1:1-27). He sat among the exiles by the river, as though bereaved, "for seven days. At the end of seven days, the Word of the Lord came to me...." (Ez. 3:15-16) In the post-exilic period, Daniel underwent ritual mourning in preparation for a night vision. He sustained "prayer and supplication with fasting and sackcloth and ashes" (Dan. 9:3). At the time of his vision, he says: "I had eaten no rich food, no meat or wine had entered my mouth, and I had not anointed myself at all, for the full three weeks" (Dan. 10:3).

Daniel gains from his ritual mourning "insight into all visions and dreams" (Dan. 1:17b). Nebuchadnezzar has a dream, and only Daniel can interpret it through a vision of the night (2:19). The God of Daniel's ancestors "reveals deep and hidden things; he knows what is in the darkness, and light dwells with him" (2:22).

The setting of Daniel's night vision is clarified as follows:

> I, Daniel, alone saw the vision; the people who were with me did not see the vision, though a great trembling fell on them, and they fled and hid themselves (10:7).
>
> So while he was speaking this word to me, I stood up trembling. He said to me, "Do not fear, Daniel...." (10:11b)
>
> "My Lord, because of the vision such pains have come upon me that I retain no strength. How can my Lord's servant talk with my Lord? For I am shaking, no strength remains in me, and no breath is left in me" (10:16b-17).

These passages indicate that Daniel suffers fear, trembling, and ecstasy, which represent the paroxysmal-epileptiform context of apocalyptic eschatology. Altogether, the visions combine into a night terror, by inhibiting Daniel's breathing and rendering him powerless. The night terror indicates a psychic distance between the visionary and a transcendent realm. The night terror signifies profound anxiety.

The psychic distance is maintained in a final vision, which employs the cross-over images of the river and the distant shore:

Then I, Daniel looked, and two others appeared, one standing on this bank of the stream and one on the other. One of them said to the man clothed in linen, who was upstream, "How long shall it be until the end of these wonders?" The man clothed in linen, who was upstream, raised his right hand and his left hand toward heaven. And I heard him swear by the one who lives forever that it would be for a time, two times, and half a time, and that when the shattering of the power of the holy people comes to an end, all these things would be accomplished (12:5-8).

Immanent consciousness is expressed by the banks of the river downstream and transcendent consciousness, as the bearer of revelation, by the river upstream. The vision promises that when the political and religious persecution of the people ends, visions will cease. The time of the end remains a secret; for it is decreed only by the Divine Warrior in heaven. The task is to endure persecution through wisdom and piety, so as to join the heavenly council after death and be radiant forever (Dan. 12:2-3).

V. JESUS' "CROSS-OVER" MINISTRY

The Gospel of Mark continues the apocalyptic eschatology of Daniel, beginning with the proclamation of John the Baptist, who cries out (*boao*) in the desert: "Prepare the way of the Lord, make his paths straight" (1:3). The proclamation is followed by John's baptism of Jesus, an event rich in shock symbolism: "And just as he was coming up out of the water, he saw the heavens torn apart and the Spirit descending like a dove on him. And a voice came from heaven, 'You are my Son, the Beloved; with you I am well pleased.'" (1:10-11) The passage contains a paroxysmal parallelism of ascent (*anabainon*) and descent (*katabainon*). Through the sacred power of water, the fiery spirit establishes a participatory bond with Jesus, making him a "bridge," as it were (Bleeker 1963, 85). The baptism is sanctified by three eschatological signs: (1) opening of the heavens; (2) descent of the Spirit; and (3) the heavenly voice.

Further, cross-over motifs appear in the healing ministry of Jesus; when he crosses the sea to the other shore, he performs a miracle (Mk. 5:21-34). The next two passages portray Jesus crossing over the waters and reenacting the same motif, as in Creation and Exodus. When evening had come, he said:

> "Let us go across to the other side." And leaving the crowd behind, they took him with them in the boat, just as he was. Other boats were with him. A great storm arose, and the waves beat into the boat, so that the boat was already being swamped. But he was in the stern, asleep on the cushion; and they woke him up and said to him, "Teacher, do you not care that we are perishing?" He woke up and rebuked the wind, and said to the sea, "Peace! Be still!" (Mk. 4:35-39)

This passage reenacts Psalm 107:29: "he made the storm be still, and the waves of the sea were hushed;" a Psalm which affirms praise and thanksgiving for deliverance from Sheol. The Greek term for rebuke (*epitimao*) is strong, and it means an aggressive discharge of energy against the demonic forces of death. As with Old Testament visions, this episode takes place at night, the time of apocalyptic revelation.

> When evening came, the boat was out on the sea, and he was alone on the land. When he saw that they were straining at the oars against an adverse wind, he came towards them early in the morning, walking on the sea. He intended to pass them by. But when they saw him walking on the sea, they thought it was a ghost and cried out; for they all saw him and were terrified. But immediately he spoke to them and said, "Take heart, it is I; do not be afraid" (Mk. 6:47-50).

The episode designates an apocalyptic situation, as revealed by the Markan code word "immediately" (*euthus*), used throughout the Gospel to stress the urgency of the end-time. The passage declares that this Jesus, who now walks on the water, is the same as the divine Spirit that swept over the dark waters at the Creation. The terror of the disciples is a natural response to the anxiety of the primal abyss.

Terror continues to build, when Jesus predicts his future suffering and death: "The Son of Man must undergo great suffering, and be rejected by the elders, the chief priest, and the scribes, and be killed, and after three days rise again" (8:31). An objective sense of danger accumulates, because Jesus' ministry collides with traditional temple religion. That Jesus intends to reform temple religion is indicated in the transfiguration, which is an apparition that correlates with the pervasive danger:

> Six days later, Jesus took with him Peter and James and John, and led them up on a high mountain apart, by themselves. And he was transfigured before them, and his clothes became dazzling white, such as no one on earth could bleach them. And there appeared to them Elijah with Moses, who were talking with Jesus. Then Peter said to Jesus, "Rabbi, it is good for us to be here; let us make three dwellings, one for you, one for Moses, and one for Elijah." He did not know what to say, for they were terrified. Then a cloud overshadowed them, and from a cloud there came a voice, "This is my Son, the Beloved; listen to him!" Suddenly when they looked around, they saw no one with them anymore, but only Jesus (Mk. 9:2-8).

The transfiguration consists of an apparition, since the verbs for "appeared" (*ophthe*) in verse four and "saw" (*eidon*) in verse eight are variants of the same term (*horao*). They denote non-sensory vision, as will be argued below in section seven. In the passage of Jesus walking on the water, cited above, the verbs for "saw" also derive from the verb (*horao*) for non-sensory vision.

Jesus is beheld, on the one hand, in relation to Moses, the prophet who had been commissioned as a "bridge" between God and the people (Deut. 18:15-18). On the other hand, Jesus is viewed in relation to Elijah, the keeper of the sacred tradition who appears in times of messianic change. Elijah had not actually died, according to tradition: "As they continued walking and talking, a chariot of fire and horses separated the two of them, and Elijah ascended in a whirlwind into heaven" (I Kgs. 2:11). Motifs of ascent and whirlwind are paroxysmal images of a shock event, that of Elijah's passing into heaven.

The mountain, on which the transfiguration occurs, is the exclusive place for revelation in the Bible. Allusions to the three dwellings (*skenas*) in verse five denote the "Tent of Meeting," where God dwelled (*skn*) with his people, during the desert sojourn between the Revelation on Sinai and the settlement (Ex. 25:8; 29:45; 36-40:35). Reenacting the image of the desert dwelling, prior to the building of the temple, is intended to renew temple worship in terms of the prophetic tradition.

The voice, approving Jesus as the "beloved son" is the same eschatological sign of the baptism, and it means that Jesus bears the prophetic tradition in the impending "Day of the Lord."

Finally, the Transfiguration stands at the center of the Gospel narrative, and in the second half the setting shifts from the mountain to the city of Jerusalem. After entering the city, Jesus goes directly to the temple, where he preaches an apocalyptic sermon (Mk. 13). Since his predictions of suffering and death lead to a confrontation with the temple authorities, his purpose for going to Jerusalem is to die and, thereby, bring about a reversal of the established order. The temple complex, including city and mountain, had been built as a "bridge" between heaven and earth (Ps. 48); but Jesus' death will overturn the sacred order of Creation.

VI. EMPTYING OF TEMPLE AND TOMB

The Gospel narrative culminates in the crucifixion of Jesus. To cope with the shame and horror of Jesus' death, Christians used selected Old Testament texts, such as (1) apocalyptic eschatology (e.g. Joel 2-3; Zech. 9-14; Dan. 7); (2) prophecies concerning Israel and her future (e.g. Isa. 6:1-9, 7); (3) Psalms of the suffering righteous and the servant songs (e.g. Ps. 22, 38, 69; Isa. 42-53); and (4) other miscellaneous passages (Weber 1979, 31).

As reported in Mark, Psalm 22 was the principal text for dealing with Jesus' death. While hanging on the cross, Jesus cries out the first verse of Psalm 22: "My God, my God, why have you forsaken me?" (Mk. 15:34b). Jesus is surely affirming the entire Psalm, since, in Jewish liturgical practice, reciting the first verse represents the entire passage. In Hebrew logic the part embodies the whole. Although the first verse of Psalm 22 laments abandonment, the rest of the Psalm declares praise. Jesus' cry of abandonment complements the cry of John the Baptist, stated at the beginning of the Gospel: "The voice of one crying out in the wilderness: 'Prepare the way of the Lord, make his paths straight'" (Mk. 1:3). In each passage the verb for crying out is the same (*boao*), a fact suggesting that abandonment prepares the way of the Lord.

To understand what Jesus thought in the face of death it is necessary to consult the remainder of Psalm 22. The Psalmist goes from the cry of abandonment to the faith of the ancestors; "Yet you are holy, enthroned on the praises of Israel. In you our ancestors trusted; they trusted, and you delivered them. To you they cried, and were saved; in you they trusted, and were not put to shame" (vs. 3-5).

The Psalmist admits he is a worm not human, scorned, despised, and mocked by "all who see me" (vs. 6-7). Nevertheless, God has been present, since his birth (vs. 9-11). He is dried up, in the dust, near death. Bulls encircle him like lions; dogs are around him (vs. 12, 16). Evil-doers divide his clothing and cast lots for it (v. 18). Yet from "you comes my praise in the great congregation; my vows I will pay before those who fear him" (v. 25). With avowal and rejoicing the Psalmist exults in the dominion of God over all the earth. Even the dead and all future generations will obey the Lord (vs. 28-31). Then the Psalm concludes with a claim of deliverance for the descendants who are yet to come.

Several decisive themes in Psalm 22 are quoted by other Gospels, which were written after Mark: abandonment (Matt. 27:46), being seen by all (Lk. 23:35), mocking (Matt. 27:39), dried up (Jn. 19:28), division of garments (Matt. 27:35; Lk. 23:34; Jn. 19:24), and trust in God (Matt. 27:43). References to the animals reflect symbolic functions known in the history of religions. The bull is a sacrificial animal, and the dog is the guardian of the dead. In the Psalm these are trace-images, suggesting the degradation of Jesus' death.

In ancient Israel the Psalms of praise represented public acts of avowal in the temple. Jesus' implied affirmation of praise was performed publically, not in the temple, but in the context of a shameful death. The overall effect of Jesus' avowal was to shatter the traditionally sharp dichotomy of tomb and temple, mourning and rejoicing. When Jesus died, "the curtain of the temple was torn in two, from top to bottom" (Mk. 15:38). The ritual dichotomy eroded, further, because the crucifixion occurred during the season of Passover and the festival of Unleavened Bread (Mk. 14:1), two festivals appointed as times of celebration and sacrifice (Num. 28:16-25; Lev. 23:5-14).

Mark portrays the essence of the crucifixion as the mystery of darkness. "When it was noon, darkness came over the whole land until three in the afternoon" (15:33). At three o'clock, Jesus cries out in abandonment, only after enduring three hours of darkness in silence. The darkness makes the death a cosmic event; for the darkness is that of the cosmic sea, the abyss of Creation (Grayston 1952). The darkness at noon recapitulates the horror and violence of Sheol (Ps. 88), the waters of which flow from the subterranean ocean of the primeval chaos (Ps. 7:12-20). During the silence of the darkness, all things return to the primal state under the power of God. When Jesus affirms Psalm 22, light returns, indicating a "re-creation" of the world. Just as darkness covered the Passover in Egypt, so is the darkness of the crucifixion a new Exodus. Through the mystery of darkness, the apocalyptic death of Jesus overturned the sacred order of Creation as represented by temple religion.

Matthew elaborated the apocalyptic nature of Jesus' death even further: "The earth shook, and the rocks were split. The tombs also were opened, and many bodies of the saints who had fallen asleep were raised" (27:52). Luke emphasizes the falling of the mountains, the darkness covering the land, and the failing of the sun's light (23:30, 44-45). Luke's image of the falling mountain comes from the prophet Hosea (10:9) and that of darkness from Amos (8:9). Altogether images of earthquake and darkness indicate that the revelation occurs in the eruptive forces of Sheol in death and grief, rather than in the temple.

John interprets Jesus' death as fulfillment of Zechariah's apocalyptic vision. In John the bystanders "look on the one whom they have pierced" (19:37), which is a quotation of Zechariah 12:10: "...when they look on the one whom they have pierced, they shall mourn for him, as one mourns for an only child, and weep bitterly over him, as one weeps over a firstborn." The historical setting for Zechariah was the rebuilding of the Temple after the Babylonian Exile, spanning a seventy year period of fasting and mourning (Zech. 8:19). By analogy, the grief for Jesus is the same as that of the exiles, who mourned until the Second Temple was rebuilt.

Matthew states that the Second Temple, built after the Exile, had become corrupted, as indicated by Judas' betrayal of Jesus for "thirty shekels of silver" (26:15). The same phrase appears in Zechariah (11:13) and signifies the corruption of the Temple treasury. The corruption of the Temple justifies the judgment in the crucifixion; since the Temple has become corrupt, it can no longer represent Creation.

The judgment of the Temple is correlated with the empty tomb episode in the Resurrection Narrative. In Mark the women go to the tomb in the morning to anoint the corpse of Jesus. Following the Old Testament custom, anointing with oil may be interpreted as an act of joy (Anderson 1991, 46). Isaiah stipulates the anointing of oil for those who have emerged from death and grief (61:3) and who obtain joy amid sorrow (35:10). By going to the tomb to anoint the body, the women intended to come to terms with their grief.

When the women arrive at the tomb, however, they discover the stone has been rolled away, and it is empty. An angel announces that Jesus has been raised from the dead and would meet them in Galilee. The women react by fleeing from the tomb in fear (*phobos*), trembling (*tromos*), and ecstasy (*ekstasis*). Mark restates the Greek text of Daniel (10), where the same three terms are found in the context of an apocalyptic night vision (Kee, et. al. 1973, 141). In both Daniel and Mark the fear, trembling, and ecstasy follow a period of mourning and anticipate a catastrophic end of the world order. In Mark the episode of the empty tomb complements the eschatological signs of the baptism. The opening of the tomb parallels that of the heavens and the ascent of Jesus corresponds to his "being raised" (*egerthe*) as expressed in an aorist passive verb with aggressive, punctiliar action. The heavenly voice of the baptism is that of the angel in the tomb. Unlike Daniel in Mark the ecstasy of the women is a vision of a new day and not the night.

VII. CRUCIFIXION AFTERIMAGE

Matthew, Luke, and John present what are commonly called resurrection appearances. After his death Jesus appears to his disciples in Galilee in Matthew (28:16-20), in Jerusalem in Luke (24:36-49), and the sea of Tiberius in John (21:1-24). The intent of these appearances is to make restitution for Jesus' death (Perrin 1977, 33). In light of the narrative context I contend that the appearances are actually apparitions and that they derive from the afterimage of Jesus' death. Frederic Myers has explained that apparitional activity builds up one week before an expected death and then from a peak gradually levels off to one year, when it ends. The New Testament describes a similar pattern but reverses the timing. The build up of apparitional activity begins with the transfiguration, as linked with Jesus' prediction of his own death and culminates in the crucifixion, probably within a one-year limit. The shock of the crucifixion releases radiant energy within a span of time that is no longer than one week. Radiance signifies the renewal of Creation and shines forever.

My argument is based upon the fact that the principal verb in the Resurrection Narrative is *horao*, which means beholding through the mind, comprehending, or recognizing. This verb correlates with the noun *harama*, which means a striking vision, whether sleeping or awake. The verb may be contrasted with *blepo*, which means seeing through the eye, watching, or noticing things.

In Matthew, the figure in the grave is an angel, who announces that the Risen Jesus will meet the women in Galilee. The context turns quickly from fear, as was the case in Mark, to great joy. The women run to tell the disciples, and together they confront Jesus in his apparitional being; and he says to them: "Greetings" (Matt. 28:9), They "seize" his feet and worship him. Following Hebrew thought, wherein the part represents the whole, feet mean the entire personality. Since the seizure lacks force, the verb (*krateo*) should be translated as apprehending, holding fast, or relating to. The apprehension of Jesus occurs apparitionally in great joy, since intense grief for his death has ended. Whereas the grief is not resolved in Mark, in Matthew it is.

Luke innovates by separating the Resurrection from the Ascension and placing the apparitions in a forty day interval between the two events. The Road to Emmaus story combines the desert tradition of hospitality (Gen. 18:1-8) with the apparitions. Two men are walking along the road and joined by a stranger, who is actually Jesus. They talk with sadness about the death of Jesus, and when they arrive at Emmaus, they break bread with the stranger, whose identity as Jesus is immediately revealed. Welcoming the stranger is a revelation of Jesus' presence and an incorporation of the deceased into the community. Welcoming the stranger coincides with the resolution of grief.

Jesus suddenly vanishes; he goes to Jerusalem and greets the disciples, who are terrified and think he is a ghost. Jesus says: "Look at my hands and my feet; see that it is I myself. Touch me and see; for a ghost does not have flesh and bones as you see that I have" (Lk. 24:39). They respond with joy, and he eats a piece of broiled fish with them. This episode is apparitional, but secondary corporeal traits inhere with the vision. The command to see (v. 39) employs *horao*, which, therefore, requires that the verb for touch (*pselopho*) be translated as "attachment" or "feeling." The second verb to see, at the end of the verse, is *theoreo*, which means "being a mental spectator," with or without open eyes.

Luke's narrative emphasizes the early Christian tradition of divine necessity. Jesus died in accordance with the scripture; his suffering and death were necessary to fulfill the Law, prophets, and the Psalms (24:44-

46), Thus, the purpose of the apparitional phase is to reveal the divine necessity.

Luke describes the Ascension as follows:

Then he led them out as far as Bethany, and, lifting up his hands, he blessed them. While he was blessing them, he withdrew from them and was carried up into heaven. And they worshiped him, and returned to Jerusalem with great joy; and they were continually in the Temple blessing God (Lk. 24:50-53).

The Ascension is an exaltation of Jesus to a state of glory or radiant being, which coincides with the release of joy and the cessation of mourning. The motif of ascent echoes that of the heavenly journey, which is the Hellenistic counterpart to the older Hebrew notion of descent into Sheol. Manifesting joy and blessing in the temple indicate that the reform of Temple religion has been accomplished.

Finally, John also deals with the resurrection apparitions in the context of Jesus' ascent to God the Father. Jesus appears first to a bereaved Mary Magdalene, saying: "Do not hold on (*haptou*) to me, because I have not yet ascended to the Father. But go to my brothers and say to them, 'I am ascending to my Father....'" (Jn. 20:17) Then he appears to his disciples at night and declares: "'Peace be with you.' After he said this, he showed them his hands and his side, then the disciples rejoiced when they saw the Lord" (Jn. 20:19b-20). This episode is followed by Jesus' conferring the Holy Spirit and apparitional signs to Thomas, the seven disciples, and to Peter.

The Johannine apparitions should be viewed in terms of the earlier farewell discourse, particularly chapter 16. Jesus acknowledges their sorrow on his departure from the world and explains that "you will weep and mourn, but the world will rejoice; you will have pain, but your pain will turn into joy" (Jn. 16:20). The anguish of grief is compared to the labor pains of birth, so that when a child is born joy replaces suffering. Hence, Jesus counsels that "you have pain now; but I will see you again, and your hearts will rejoice, and no one will take your joy from you" (16:22).

Jesus encourages detachment from him and from the world on the grounds that sorrow turns into joy. Therefore, Jesus' command to Mary Magdalene must be interpreted as: "Do not cling to me," which is one of the meanings of *haptou*. The passage reveals a profound insight into the dynamics of grief. To cling, or hold on to the earthly Jesus is to become depressed and to prolong the pain and suffering of the crucifixion. Refusing to cling prevents depression and allows Jesus to ascend to the Father, to absent himself from the world. With the absence of Jesus, a new power is conferred, namely the turning of sorrow into joy. The capacity for joy signifies both the stark reality of the crucifixion and the exaltation of Jesus.

VIII. APOCALYPTIC TRANSFIGURATION

Ever since the age of the prophets, the world had been understood as the arena, where the Divine Warrior fought the inimical power of death. As the supreme adversary, death had ruled the world, holding humankind in bondage, but with the crucifixion, early Christians believed that God had defeated death decisively. The entire order of the world had been overturned, as signified by the emptying of the tomb and Temple.

Despite the victory on the cross, the expected "Day of the Lord" had not yet arrived. It would come as a day of judgment at the end of the world, when the wrath of God would shatter all traces of death forever. The earliest theologian, the apostle Paul, believed that evil would expand before the end until it reached a climax, at which point God would intervene and subdue all hostile, demonic forces. Paul's apocalyptic vision is clearly expressed in II Thessalonians, according to which the signs of intensified evil are rebelliousness, lawlessness, and delusion (2:2-3, 9-10). For Paul evil is an innate tendency, which is driven by the power of death (Rom. 6:23; 8:2; I Cor. 15:56).

With the judgment, the order of death and evil will be totally destroyed. This order consists of a physical continuum linked to humankind, as exemplified by the phrase "flesh and blood." At judgment a spiritual body will be disinhibited by flesh and blood, and it too will intensify into an invisible, transpersonal community. Within the spiritual body all the living and all the dead will be changed (I Cor. 15:51; Phil. 3:21). The time of the judgment remains unknown; for the "Day of the Lord" will come like a thief in the night (I Thes. 5:2).

The same apocalyptic vision was carried to an even higher level of power in the Revelation to John. The later chapters narrate the destruction of Babylon, which is the demonic symbol of Rome, that has been thrown into the sea by the mighty angel (18:21). The sea is the dark and formless void of Creation, the primal abyss (Gen. 1:2). As the heavenly multitudes rejoiced, suddenly a rider on a white horse appeared, one "called Faithful and True," whose eyes were like flames of fire, who judged and made war (19:11-12). The rider on the white horse is the Christ, the Word of God, who conquers the forces of evil and throws them alive into Gehenna, the lake of fire burning with sulphur.

Then the angel descends from heaven, captures Satan the Devil, serpent and dragon, and throws him into the pit or Sheol, where he is bound for a thousand years. After that time, Satan ascends to fight, but once again he is slain by the fire and cast into the burning water. The dead are then judged before the heavenly throne, according to the Book of Life (20:12), which is a record of human actions (Dan. 7:10). Those omitted from the book are thrown into the lake of fire to suffer the second death. These striking paroxysmal images of ascent and descent, fire and water are symbolizations of violent death.

Then John "saw a new heaven and a new earth; for the first heaven and the first earth had passed away, and the sea was no more" (21:1). John's vision signifies the final conquest of the primeval order and chaos, out of which a new order emerges. John "saw the holy city, the new Jerusalem, coming down out of heaven from God, prepared as a bride adorned for her husband" (21:2). The wedding motif inaugurates a time of joy and the end of grief: "he will wipe every tear from their eyes. Death will be no more; mourning and crying and pain will be no more, for the first things have passed away" (21:3-4).

The holy city is a radiant jewel, as bright and as clear as crystal, a symbol of fundamental reality. The Temple is absent, and, as in the ancient desert period, God dwells directly with the people in glory. The radiant light dissolves the primal distinction between day and night. Within the city flows the river of the water of life, in contrast to the holy water of the Temple, taken from the primal ocean. Flowing water symbolizes atonement and regeneration of the order of the world.

With great visionary power John bequeathed to the ages a crucifixion afterimage, whose radiant light shines forever within the transfigured universe. In the centuries yet to come the vision of radiant being would turn death into life and sorrow into joy. Empowered by this vision, early Christians received the courage to face sorrow directly.

CHAPTER EIGHT:
FORMATION OF PONTIFICAL
SELFHOOD

I. REVERSAL OF THE WORLD ORDER

The early Christian community believed that the crucifixion of Jesus had been a turning point in history. Early Christians understood Jesus' death as an active defeat of the demonic force of death that had governed the world, the stars, and the planets. By destroying the rule of death, the order of the world had been overturned. This conviction was attested in the collapse of the dichotomy of Sheol and the Temple in the drama of the crucifixion. Consequently, after the crucifixion of Jesus, death was no longer feared as alien and demonic but was greeted joyously. Similarly, sudden death had been interpreted as a result of evil intentions; but since the shock of the crucifixion had become a revelation of divine love, sudden death was no longer dreaded either. Early Christians affirmed these convictions through baptism, in which they identified with the death of the Christ (Rom. 6:10-11).

The reversal of the world order was confirmed by a new burial practice. In the pre-Christian world the dead were buried outside the city, usually alongside a road. Luke 7:12 illustrates this custom, stating that "a man who had died was being carried out" for burial. In contrast, with the arrival of the Christian era the dead would be buried within the city, in collective and unmarked graves, and frequently in Church yards (Ariès 1981, 24-36). Since the crucifixion had conquered the terror of death, the dead were no longer feared; and so burial within city walls made the dead familiar and no longer threatening. Exceptions were granted for those who became excommunicated, prisoners, and social outcasts. Nevertheless, the Christian community embraced the living and the dead as members of one family. This change of burial custom did not take place quickly but evolved gradually until finished about the year 500 C.E.. A breakthrough occurred in the fourth century, when Roman persecutions ceased and Christianity became legally established, thus making public funerals possible. Christian funerals celebrated death with Psalms of thanksgiving and joy (Pss. 23, 32, 115, 116).

The principal bearers of the new view of death were the martyrs. In particular, the martyrdom of Stephen reenacted the crucifixion of Jesus as murder of the righteous one (Acts 7:52). After his arrest, Stephen delivered a speech retelling the history of the patriarchs in Genesis and proclaiming that the "God of glory appeared to our ancestor Abraham" as well as Moses and others (Acts 7). Stephen therefore identified the prophets as both ancestors and bearers of the Christian revelation. By incorporating the prophets within the historical community, they became familiar figures in the dynamic tradition.

Meanwhile, the Johannine and Pauline theologies informed the martyrdom of Ignatius of Antioch (Meinhold 1980, 154). Ignatius was Pauline in making his own suffering and death an imitation of Christ, and he was Johannine in renouncing the world. Martyrdom is the occasion to separate from finite existence and to participate in the exalted Christ. The martyr acquires a true being by participating in the exalted Christ in joy. Ignatius' martyrdom changed the meaning of the eucharist from a recollection of the body and blood of Jesus to the "medicine of immortality" (*pharmakon athanasias*). In light of the Greek phrase immortality is understood as "deathlessness" rather than as survival of the soul (to the Ephesians 20:2).

Ignatius describes death in terms of shock suffering:

> Indulge me in what is most expedient for me. I know now I am beginning to be a disciple. Let no one visible or invisible be jealous that I might obtain Jesus Christ. Fire and crucifixion, struggles with wild beasts, mutilation, torture, scattering of bones, mangling of limbs, grinding of the entire body, evil torture of the Devil, let them come upon me, provided that I attain Jesus Christ. (to the Romans 5:3, my trans.)

This statement, so rich in paroxysmal imagery, portrays dying as an ecstatic seizure, in which Ignatius surrenders himself in order to conquer evil. Restitution is achieved in his suffering, and death is disclosed as a passage to a new, transfigured being. The combination of joy and willingness to die exemplifies the biblical ideal of radiance as normative.

II. CRITIQUE OF DREAM AND VISION

Bearing a new vision of death, early Christians developed their tradition by means of dreams and visions, as in the times of the patriarchs and the prophets. For example, Peter was travelling, and he became hungry. Suddenly, he fell into a trance and beheld the heavens opening:

> ...and something like a large sheet coming down, being lowered to the ground by its four corners. In it were all kinds of four-footed creatures and reptiles and birds of the air. Then he heard a voice saying, "Get up Peter; kill and eat." But Peter said, "By no means, Lord; for I have never eaten anything that is profane or unclean." The voice said to him again, a second time, "What God has made clean, you must not call profane" (Acts 10:10-15).

The text indicates that the vision appeared three times, which would support the argument, in chapter five, that a three fold manifestation of a dream is a resolution of conflict. Three men arrive, and the Holy Spirit commands Peter to go with them, preaching to all regardless of religious affiliation. The vision reconciles Jewish-Christian conflicts over food laws and divisions over sacred and profane customs.

Similarly, Paul receives a vision of the night: "There stood a man of Macedonia pleading with him and saying. 'Come over to Macedonia and help us'" (Acts 16:9). Paul responded to the call, crossed over to Macedonia, and consequently took Christianity to Europe. Sometime later, when threatened with opposition in Corinth, Paul had another vision in which God said: "'Do not be afraid, but speak and do not be silent, for I am with you....'" (Acts 18:9-10a)

Ironically, by the second century early Christians became suspicious of dreams, and they rejected them as sources of religious knowledge. Suspicion of the dream would become a permanent trend, lasting well into the Middle Ages (Le Goff 1984, 177). At the same time, early Christians began to consider visions more critically, rather than taking them automatically. They raised questions, so as to ascertain the validity of visions. Are they authentic? Are they true? Do they come from God?

Ernst Benz explains that the critique of dreams and visions had two motivations (1968, 23). One was that dreams belonged to the mystery religions, divination, oracles, and particularly, the Asclepius cult of faith healing. The other was that the struggling Christian community, in order to distinguish itself from those Greco-Roman movements, had to reject the dream and become more critical of the vision. Hence, the Christian critique of dream and vision was the beginning of Western psychology.

Exploring these two reasons further would reveal more clearly the profound implications of the Christian critique for the psychology of death. First, Christianity rejected dreams as sources of revelation, because they were associated with divination. The term divination derives from the Latin verb *divinari*, which means "to predict." Predicting is related to the notion of the divine (*divinus*) in the sense that a god possesses one in ecstasy, enabling one to grasp hidden truths. The act of speaking in the ecstatic state is called prophecy. Generally, divination refers to what, following Frederic Myers, is called clairvoyance and telepathy, retrocognition and precognition.

According to Cicero, divination comprised two types, depending on the method (*De Divinatione* 1:11; 2:26). One was artificial, and it was conducted with entrails, prodigies, lightning, augury, astrology, and lots. The other was natural, and it obtained from dreams and ecstatic states. With respect to natural divination and prophecy, Cicero reported the belief of the Stoic Posidonius concerning the mind during unconscious states. The fresh new translation by Georg Luck is cited (1985, 274):

When, in sleep, the mind is separated from the companionship of the body and is not in touch with it, it remembers the past, sees the present, foresees the future. The body of the sleeper lies as if he were dead, but his mind is alert and active. This is true to a much higher degree after death, when the mind has left the body altogether; therefore, when death approaches, the mind is much more divine. For those who are seriously, critically ill see the approach of death; therefore, they have visions of the dead....(Cicero, *De Div.* 1:63)

This position of Posidonius presupposed, among Stoic philosophers, the image of Socrates facing a death sentence: "Now I wish to make a prophecy to you, my fellow citizens who have sentenced me to death, for I have now reached the point where human beings are particularly apt to deliver prophecies--shortly before they die" (**Apology** 39C1, Luck trans.). Some Greek philosophers, notably Aristotle, believed that the soul could achieve comparable prophetic powers in epilepsy (Temkin 1971, 157). As described in chapter one, the same connection between facing a death sentence, enhanced psychic ability, and epilepsy was made by Dostoevsky.

In contrast to the image of Socrates, as preserved by Stoicism, Christianity regarded the image of the dying Jesus as normative. The earliest Gospel tradition did not emphasize Jesus' prophetic powers but, rather, it rejoiced in God, despite his apparent abandonment, through Psalm 22 (Mk. 15:34).

However, a much more controversial use of dreams, from the perspective of Christianity, occurred in the faith healing cult of Asclepius. Asclepius was a revered figure in Greek mythology. His father was the god Apollo, and his mother the human Coronis. He became a renown healer, who even had the reputation of preventing death and restoring the dead to life. Asclepius travelled from city to city, walking with a staff and accompanied by a dog. In the fourth century B.C.E. a sanctuary of Asclepius was built at Epidaurus, where the sacred serpent became associated with the healer. Devotees went to the shrine, made sacrifices, slept in a dormitory, and sooner or later beheld Asclepius in a dream. He would flare up, as light out of darkness, and prescribe a cure to the dreamer. The dream was an epiphany of the supernatural; and upon awakening one would rejoice in the power of the rising sun.

In the classical age of the city-state the Asclepius cult remained private; but during the Hellenistic and Roman periods, Asclepius evolved as a major deity, whose cult centered in Pergamon. In the second century of the Christian era Asclepius was called the "god of Pergamon" and celebrated as a savior figure, with whom the people could establish a personal relationship. The rise of Asclepius was due to his link with the Caesars and to his popularity in the Roman army. The Roman orator Aelius Aristides proclaimed the power of Asclepius to be great, good, and universal, the ruler and guide of all things. In his **Speaking to**

Asclepius (355.4) Aristides declares that healing occurs in the words (*Lalia*) of the god (Habicht 1969, 13).

The Asclepius cult deviated from the rational, naturalistic approach to medicine established by Hippocrates in the fifth century B.C.E.. The Hippocratic text *Regimen* states that dreams are useful in diagnosing disease (IV). However, in his commentary Robert Joly points out that Hippocrates does not support divination, because the dream is a symptom of the present state of the body and not a means of prediction (1967, xxii).

The claims of the Asclepius cult came into direct conflict with Christianity, wherein the God of Abraham is the ruler of all things and Jesus is recognized as "Savior of the World" (Jhn. 4:42). In the second century a struggle broke out in Pergamon between the followers of Jesus and Asclepius. Many Christians had been martyred in Pergamon. Evidence of this conflict comes from the Revelation, where the angel gives a message to the church of Pergamon: "I know where you are living, where Satan's throne is" (Rev. 2:13a). The throne of Satan is the Asclepius shrine at Pergamon. This is proven by the image of the god, sitting on a throne with a serpent, on coins excavated by archeologists (Rengstorf 1953, 28). As early as the reign of Emperor Domitian, the image of Asclepius began to appear on the coins of the city. Domitian ruled between 81-96 C.E., when Revelation was written. The serpent of Asclepius was also a coat of arms for Pergamon and its identification with Satan meant that the cult was the dragon of the apocalypse: "The great dragon was thrown down, that ancient serpent, who is called the Devil and Satan, the deceiver of the whole world—he was thrown down to the earth...." (Rev. 12:9)

The Christian struggle against Asclepius was also against Rome, the sponsor of the god's cult. Rome acquired the Asclepius cult as early as 293 B.C.E. in order to secure healings during the plague. In **From the Founding of the City** Livy reports that a group brought the sacred serpent from Epidaurus and sailed on a boat up the Tiber River to the island, where a temple to Asclepius was built (X. XLVVI.7). The Tiber island is shaped like a boat, and in contemporary Rome the Church of San Bartolomeo stands on the original site of the Asclepius shrine. The walls of the church still show traces of the serpent and the staff emblems.

Locating the Asclepius cult on the Tiber River island had profound implications for cultural and religious history. During the archaic period of Rome, *Pontifex Maximus* built the first bridge (*Pons Sublicius*) over the Tiber River and near the island. *Pontifex Maximus* was the supreme priest-engineer of Rome who could build the bridge because he knew how to appease the river deity, namely, by making sacrifices. The Roman emperors took over the title of *Pontifex Maximus* as deified figures, and they held it until 379 C.E.. Thereafter, the title belonged to the popes as the exclusive bridge between heaven and earth. However, with the papacy the term *Pontifex* meant one who makes a pathway into unknown regions and defends against danger (Bleeker 1963, 184).

When construction of the Vatican was completed in the sixteenth century, the site chosen overlooked the *Pons Sublicius*. This meant that the pontificate would forever conquer the Devil. For in the classical age the archaic river deity was associated with the Devil (Knight 1953, 851). The Book of Revelation had not only identified Asclepius as Satan but had also linked him to the river (12:15). Thus, the conquest of Satan facilitated salvation, by providing a bridge to heaven through the Roman Catholic papacy.

III. VISION AND THE BRIDGE

Since the Roman Catholic pontificate understood itself in terms of the bridge symbol, it is my contention that Szondi's theory of the pontifical ego represents the normative conception of selfhood in classical Western civilization. The rise of the papacy coincided with the Christian critique of dream and vision; so the concept of pontifical selfhood also represents the origin of Western psychology.

My contention opposes the view of Carl Jung, who rejected the Christian conception of selfhood as normative on the assumption that Medieval Christianity was too primitive. He meant that classical Christianity lacked a realistic appreciation of evil, because it defined evil as the absence of good. In contrast, Jung believed that evil is a radical force that can no longer be conceived as the absence of good; for good and evil are relativized (1961, 329). Both good and evil need to be integrated psychically in order to achieve self-realization. Theologically, such an integration requires the incorporation of the Devil into the Godhead, along with the Father, Son, and Holy Spirit, thus turning the Trinity into a quaternity. Since quaternity represents the logical structure of the mandala, Jung interpreted the cross as a mandala. The cross fits the mandala-quaternity structure, because it has four points. Recovering the cross as an authentic mandala in Christianity would compensate for the one-sided Trinitarian theology that split evil off from the ultimate ground of the psyche.

Jung's interpretation is questionable theologically and historically. First his identification of the cross with the mandala fits only a limited time and place but cannot refer to classical Christianity. An identification of the cross with the mandala did appear in Central Asia in the eighth century C.E., when Nestorian Christians of the Eastern Church travelled eastward along the "Silk roads" and interacted with Buddhist communities and Shamanism. In Nestorian theology the cross represents the risen, transfigured Christ who has conquered death and fulfilled all mystery. The Nestorians made a sharp contrast between the exalted Christ and the suffering, dying Jesus, hanging on the cross, as proclaimed in the Western Church.

In a Nestorian inscription at Sianfu (781 C.E.), the cross is portrayed as a cosmic sign that reenacts the creation of the world: God "sets the cross to determine the four directions of heaven" (Klimkeit 1980, 67). Similarly, in a Chinese inscription of the thirteenth century the cross is "a symbol of the four quarters, above and below." These inscriptions prove the cross to be a mandala in the sense that it coordinates the four fold dimension of the universe in a spatial-mythical system. Cross and universe share a microcosmic-macrocosmic relationship, respectively. However, the inscriptions do not provide evidence of the cross as an integration of good and evil, as Jung's position requires.

Second, Jung fails to grasp the fundamental truth of biblical and classical Christianity, which is transmitted in the Western tradition of the "wooden cross" as opposed to the "light cross" of the Nestorians. Normative Christianity claims the expiation of evil in the crucifixion of Jesus. This means that the demonic dread of death has been defeated and the order of the world overturned. Jung does not discuss the concept of restitution or atonement; for evil cannot be conquered, since it is relative to the good. Good and evil comprise a logically equivalent polarity.

One of Jung's targets is St. Augustine, who explains that Christianity seeks freedom through love and liberation from sin, death, and evil (**City of God** V:18). Augustine faithfully represents the intent of the atonement doctrine in the theology of the Western Church. Admittedly, Augustine defines evil as the absence of the good, but this definition presupposes the insight that humankind acts in a defective manner because of freedom. God is Being-itself, unchangeable and eternal, who encompasses evil as nonbeing. While Jung does not fully appreciate the Christian conception of atonement, his concern that radical evil be acknowledged is certainly consistent with experience and will be developed later in Martin Luther's theology.

In contrast to Jung's position Szondi's theory of the pontifical ego represents the normative conception of selfhood in classical Christianity. To support my contention, in the remainder of this section, I sketch four components of pontifical selfhood and briefly summarize them as follows: (1) psychic expansion from the bodily ego to a transpersonal level of being ("p"); (2) complementary range of practical decision-making, realistic adaptation, and sense of possession ("k"); (3) principle of restitution or liberation; and (4) experience of projective-participation, integration, and transcendence.

(1) In the classical era the meaning of vision changed from that of a dream equivalent, as in the Bible, to that of the otherworld journey (Dinzelbacher 1978, 120, 124-125). Hence, a vision was the release of the soul from the body and movement to another place or time, whether over or under the earth. Visions come in states of ecstasy, either when sleeping or awake; and ordinary waking consciousness recedes into the background. The recipient falls asleep or into a trance and seems to be dead. He begins a heavenly journey, escorted by an angel or saint. He travels to a destination and, upon arriving, the visionary beholds paradise or the heavenly Jerusalem, purgatory with fire and water, or hell. The journey crosses a concrete landscape with pleasant, enjoyable places. The guide explains the meaning of the locations. Images of the other world, such as fields, rivers, or bridges, stand out in the foreground as means of crossing over to the beyond, which is a sacred space. The encounter with the beyond is so intense that it alters the visionaries' life. As stated in chapter four, the vision has a mandate or calling, which provides the change.

The vision befalls one as a shock event; the visionary is passive and startled. The visionary tends to be male, either priest, monk, or layman. The vision is a unique, once-in-a-lifetime event. Recipients of the vision emerge from trance, after which they are regarded as normal. Visions are not psychopathological.

This model of vision as otherworld journey persisted, virtually unchanged, from the sixth to the thirteenth century in the European Middle Ages. It occurred mainly in Nordic-Germanic, Anglo-Saxon, and French cultures. Visions were written in Latin manuscripts and transmitted within their respective intellectual traditions. Their prototypes were the Myth of Er and the Dream of Scipio in Greco-Roman tradition, and the heavenly journeys of Fourth Ezra and First Enoch in the Hebrew.

(2) During the era of the vision literature, a transition from synthetic to analytic speech took place in Western Europe and the Eastern Mediterranean areas. Classical Greek and Latin had synthetic forms in accord with the rational and harmonious quality of civilized antiquity. Classical synthesis reduces events to momentary actions without extension in time or relation. Toward the end of the Roman Empire, the synthesis of language began to disintegrate. For example, in Greek the infinitive disappeared, so that the future had to be expressed by the phrase "in order that" (*hina*) and a dependent clause. This trend had already begun in I John of the New Testament. The loss of the infinitive in Greek paralleled the absence of the infinitive in Semitic languages. This indicates that the Middle East was a self-contained cultural unit from the break up of Rome, throughout Byzantine civilization, and up to modern times. The infinitive is still lacking in Modern Greek.

At the same time, in Latin the future was conceived with the auxiliary verb "to have," and it would be represented by an act of will, by domination or possession (Borkenau 1981, 150). The use of auxiliary verbs indicates a will to control the physical world, both spatially and temporally. By the sixth century C.E. auxiliaries had replaced the simple future. In a parallel development the personal pronoun "I" entered Latin from Old Norse. The personal pronoun moved from Scandinavia to England and finally to France. The sense of "I" joined that of "having" in order to express control of the future and of the environment.

The changes in Latin corresponded to the migrations of Saxons, Irish, and Vikings. Their cultural legacies included mythic visions of the world, cross-over symbols (e.g. the bridge), and otherworld journeys. Prehistoric art in these areas featured the Celtic cross, wheel, and boat symbols, particularly in tombs, as described in chapter three. The implication of these facts is that Northwestern European cultures created the ego, after envisioning an otherworld journey beyond the self. Thus, the controlling power of the self and the participatory power, Szondi's "k" and "p" principles, respectively, came together as a result of these migrations.

(3) The era of migrations, following the decline of Rome, also brought serious social upheavals. Middle Europe lacked central authority because the seat of the empire had been transferred from Rome to Constantinople in 330 C.E.. The political division between Constantinople and Rome corresponded to the respective changes in Greek and Latin. Without a central political authority Europe was besieged by blood feud; personal and tribal vengeance replaced Roman law. In this crisis the Roman Catholic Church emerged as the only system of authority, and it enforced discipline by means of public confession and penance. The system of public penance carried on the practice of the New Testament (I Cor. 5:3-5) and of early Christianity (*Didache*).

During the fourth and fifth centuries, monks in Ireland and Wales began to write guidelines for moral discipline in terms of private and secret confession and penance. Known as the Celtic Penitentials, these texts were used by monks to absolve sin, and they could be repeated. Implied in the new penitential system was a sense of individual privacy, a factor facilitating the spread of the personal pronoun "I." Gradually, the Celtic Penitentials were taken to Europe by Irish missionaries. Since the continent was ravaged by violence and social unrest, the penitentials became useful means of expiation. At first, the continental church tried to suppress the new private penitentials and retain the older public system of penance. However, by 656 C.E. the Celtic practices were recognized and by 1075 fully established in the church.

Throughout the Middle Ages both the public and private confessionals co-existed. The public system comprised two forms. One was solemn, unrepeatable, and conducted by the Bishop. The other involved the penitential pilgrimage as expiation for such crimes as homicide and incest (Vogel 1964, 117-128). Normally, a murderer went into exile for ten years, wearing chains or walking nude. The penitential pilgrimage presupposed the exile of Cain (Gen. 4:12-14) as punishment for murder, and it functioned as an earthly counterpart to the heavenly journey.

Walking penitential pilgrimages created the need for more bridges. By the eleventh century bridge-building became just as prominent as church-building. Peter Dinzelbacher and Harold Kleinschmidt have shown that in Medieval folk traditions bridge-building was an extension of penance (1984, 255-257). To give money for the building or maintenance of a bridge was the same as giving alms or performing charitable works. Between the eleventh and the fifteenth centuries, the bridge became a symbol of the penitential journey after death. Just as we must cross bridges in this world, so must we do the same in the next. Crossing the heavenly bridge was a test of one's deeds in life. In the high Middle Ages the notion that donations to a bridge remitted punishment in the next world complied with the principle of restitution.

(4) The motif of crossing the bridge informed the Medieval vision literature, and the classical image of the bridge came from Gregory the Great, who was Pope between 540-604. About 593 Gregory wrote his **Dialogues**, which portray the bridge in book four. The **Dialogues** contain miracle stories of the Italian fathers, narrated in terms of the biblical "holy men," which are intended to provide inspiration for the struggling church long after the age of martyrdom (Petersen 1984, 24, 27, 130). Although there were political and linguistic divisions, Gregory drew upon a common theological tradition, largely shaped by the spirituality of the Eastern Church. Central to the Eastern tradition was the living man of God, whose radiance represented the beauty of holiness.

Gregory begins the **Dialogues** by admitting his depression over the world situation specifically invasions, epidemics, and schisms; and he expresses his mood with a cross-over image:

> I am tossed about on the waves of a heavy sea, and my soul is like a helpless ship buffeted by raging winds. When I recall my former way of life, it is as though I were once more looking back toward land and sighing as I beheld the shore. It only saddens me the more to find that, while flung about by the mighty waves that carry me along, I can hardly catch sight any longer of the harbor I have left (I:1, Zimmerman, trans.).

For Gregory the world is an abyss, in which humankind suffers life as an exile. In the Fall Adam lost the inner light, through which the joy of heaven is known. Only in the ecstasy of a spiritual vision, purified by faith, might the world be envisaged in a ray of light. The mind has its own image-making capacity, whose power is enhanced by dramatic death experiences, that is, by miracles.

As evidence of the mind's visionary power, Gregory recalls how Benedict saw the soul of Germanus being carried out of his body in the fire of the night (I:35). Germanus died forty miles away from where

Benedict was living. Benedict "beheld a flood of light shining down from above more brilliant than the sun;" and "the whole world was gathered up before his eyes in what appeared to be a single ray of light." Gregory emphasizes that Benedict's vision took place at midnight, a deep, dark, uncanny time. Thus, he reenacts the biblical tradition of the night vision, following Psalm 119:62 (Steidle 1971, 301).

The miracle was a cosmic vision, which in modern times, after Frederic Myers, would be called clairvoyance. Commenting on the miracle, Gregory explains:

> All creation is bound to appear small to a soul that sees the Creator. Once it beholds a little of His light, it finds all creatures small indeed. The light of holy contemplation enlarges and expands the mind in God until it stands above the world. In fact, the soul that sees Him rises even above itself, and as it is drawn upward in His light all its inner powers unfold. Then, when it looks down from above, it sees how small everything is that was beyond its grasp before.

Gregory's key observation that the mind "enlarges and expands" conforms to the gift of prophecy, as described above by Greek philosophers. Whereas, philosophy made the doomed Socrates the agent of prophecy, Gregory makes the living holy man the bearer of this gift. Gregory also learned of the discernment of the spirit and the gift of prophecy from the Eastern Church (Petersen 1984, 167). The holy man is capable of discerning the divine light, which compresses the world into a point.

Many of the miracles described by Gregory correspond to those reported in twentieth century clinical literature. For example, in the hour of death, the saints suffer neither fear nor agony, while they hear the sounds of celestial singing. Sometimes fragrant odors spread in the milieu of the dying (IV:15). When two monks were killed during the Lumbard invasion, their disembodied souls sang Psalms in search of expiation and terrified their killers. Gregory even states that the dying soul can predict the future. As Gerontius was dying, he named other monks who would also die (IV:27).

The image of the bridge appears in the context of a near-death experience of a Roman soldier:

He saw a river whose dark waters were covered by a mist of vapors that gave off an unbearable stench. Over the river was a bridge. It led to pleasant meadows beyond, covered by green grass and dotted with richly scented flowers. These meadows seemed to be the gathering places for people dressed in white robes. The fragrant odors pervading the region were a delight for all who lived there. Everyone had his own dwelling, which gleamed with brilliant light. One house of magnificent proportions was still under construction and the bricks used were made of gold (IV:37).

Gregory emphasizes that the images of the vision are not literal but symbolic. Bridge and river symbolize the narrow way to eternal life, as told in the Bible (Matt. 7:14). The abyss symbolizes carnal desire, which is punishable by sulphur and fire (Gen. 19:24). At the end of the world a cleansing fire produces different kinds of burning, according to one's moral and spiritual character.

Finally, Gregory declares that visions of the night reveal the spiritual world in contrast to the transitoriness of life. The world resembles a dark night, which merges with the light of the next world, in the same way that darkness recedes at dawn. Visions of the night are distinguished from dreams, which are associated with divination and which have six kinds of causes: full or empty stomach, illusion, thought and illusion, revelation, or thought and revelation (IV:50). Since the sources of dreams are so diverse, they should be analyzed critically. Thus, Gregory carries on the Christian trend of de-emphasizing dreams, while at the same time he elevates the night vision to the level of apocalyptic spirituality. Through his apocalyptic vision Gregory establishes the bases of pontifical selfhood: projective-participation by crossing the bridge; integration by spanning this world and the next; and transcendence by reaching the other world.

IV. RESTITUTION AND THE BRIDGE

In the concept of pontifical selfhood the exaltation of the participatory self is made possible by the experience of atonement or liberation. In the vision literature, generally, the bridge symbol directly correlates with the function of restitution. To illustrate this function a few examples of additional visions of the bridge are considered, using material in the classic study of Howard Patch (1980). The first example is the Vision of Sunniulf, written in 575 and reported by Gregory of Tours. It emphasizes the narrowness of the bridge and the drowning of sinners, motifs underdeveloped in the **Dialogues** of Gregory the Great:

> Sunniulf was led to a certain fiery river at the shore of which people were gathering like bees at a beehive, and some were submerged to the waist, some to the armpits, and some to the chin. Over the river was a bridge so narrow that there was scarcely room for one foot on it. On the other side was a large white house. Sunniulf asks the meaning of all this and is told that those religious who are careless of the discipline of their flock fall from the bridge and those who are strict pass over it safely to the house (98).

In the eighth century vision of Wenlock, he

> sees a pitchy river boiling and flaming, over which was placed a timber for a bridge. Over this the holy and glorious souls strove to pass. Some went securely, others slipped and fell into the tartarean stream. Some were wholly submerged in the flood, others to the knees, some to the middle of the body, and some to the ankles. All eventually came out of the fire rendered bright and clean to ascend the other shore. Beyond the river were walls shining with splendor great in length and height—the heavenly Jerusalem. Evil spirits were plunged into the fiery pits (101).

Finally, in the twelfth century legend of Saint Patrick's Purgatory, Owen enters a cave after fifteen days of fasting and prayer. He proceeds through various planes, until arriving at the top of a mountain, where he

> sees a fiery pit, and a broad fiery river filled with demons, over which is a slippery bridge so narrow that one could not stand on it and so high it makes one dizzy to look downwards. Owen, however, calls on the Holy Name, and the bridge becomes broader as he passes over it. At length he reaches Paradise, which is surrounded by a high wall, one gate of which is adorned with the precious stones and metals (115).

Citing these three texts illustrates the fact that, in addition to Gregory's vision, the symbolism of the bridge in the Middle Ages conformed to that of the Chinvat Bridge in Zoroastrianism and its Persian sources. The bridge becomes wide for the righteous and narrow for the unrighteous. Psychologically, the wide bridge symbolizes the making of restitution in one's life and the achieving of transcendent participation in the next world. The narrow bridge symbolizes the failure of restitution and participation.

Death is symbolized as a journey, and water represents one of the obstacles along the way. This symbol reenacts the ancient belief that rivers are universal means of organizing territorial boundaries (Zalesky 1987, 62). The image of the river of fire means that restitution may be achieved at the boundaries of existence and in the depths of life.

V. DISINTEGRATION OF THE BRIDGE

The foregoing sketch of the Medieval bridge reveals that the psychological principles of restitution and participation were active in the symbol. To cross the bridge is to unify the psychic opposites of life and death, light and darkness, good and evil and, thereby, to become liberated and whole. These two principles were necessary in light of historical conditions. Between the end of the Roman Empire and the beginning of the Middle Ages, widespread killing took place in Europe. Viking invaders overran the continent, and, in the absence of the Roman army, kings and territorial princes fought in self-defense. There was a general feeling that the Viking invasions were God's punishment for the sins of the nobility (Rosenwein 1971, 149). In the same period sporadic outbreaks of the plague also occurred. The high mortality rates from invasions and epidemic undermined the early Christian claim of the conquest of death. In this era, known as the "Dark Ages," the Christian reversal of the world order had become undone, releasing latent forces of aggression and killing. These could be denied because the killing was to protect the Church.

Ironically, formation of pontifical selfhood, begun by Gregory the Great and sustained by other visions, created a movement toward a greater synthesis of psychic antitheses, which gave rise to the high civilization of the Middle Ages. The shift from the "Dark Ages" to the Middle Ages occasioned a change from a denial of death to an acceptance of death. The acceptance released a new vitality within Medieval society (Borkenau 1981, 78-82).

The movement toward a Medieval synthesis began about the eleventh century, primarily in the reforms of the Cluny monastery. Monasteries had been established by the lay nobility to atone for the pervasive guilt over the killing of invaders during the "Dark Ages." The monks at Cluny offered intercession for the nobility, who feared the apparent end of the world, judgment, and damnation. The liturgy at Cluny included prayer vigils, masses for the dead, and, in particular, seven collects sung for the dead at matins. In 1083 the monk Ulrich described the seven collects as follows:

> the first [collect] is for brothers who died recently...the second is for the anniversary [of the death] of those named at chapter; the third is for all our dead familiars (*familiaribus*); the fourth for dead brothers; the fifth for all buried in our cemetery; the sixth for our sisters and other female familiars; the seventh for all departed faithful (Cited in Rosenwein 1971, 140).

The collects comprised Psalm 50 as well as four additional Psalms called *familiares* (Pss. 31, 69, 85, 141), which pray for deliverance from enemies, persecution, evil and for restoration of divine favor. The collects named the dead as individuals and as members of a household for the first time in the Christian era. When the dead were buried inside the city, they were not identified as individuals. Conceiving of the dead in personal terms, i.e. as familiars, employed the Latin term for family or household (*familiaris*), and it represented an original insight into the familial unconscious (*Die familiäre Unbewusste*), as discovered by Szondi in contemporary psychiatry.

Monastic reform encouraged the contemplation of death in two distinct forms. One was the contempt of the world, due to its poverty, powerlessness, and pervasive sinfulness. The other was a direct contemplation of death as directed by the well-known Latin phrase, *Memento Mori*, which meant: "Remember, you will die." These dual practices were originally created as meditative techniques for young priests, who were concerned with the hour of death and with living a proper life in preparation for dying. "The uncertainty about the hour of death was a stimulus to constant wakefulness and fear for mortal sins, which alone might separate us from the vision of God" (Rudolf 1957,

11). Preparation for death entailed maintaining the faith, the right will, withstanding temptations of sin and evil, and taking the sacraments of the Church.

Contemplating death aimed to arouse a moral consciousness, so as to transfer one's ego onto a higher level of spiritual being. These moral and psychological tasks were facilitated by a cohesive, stratified society, grounded in the natural law and the righteousness of God. The God of justice governs the lawful universe according to the principles of proportionate punishment and mercy for exceptional cases. The task of the person is to live in hope of reward or dread of punishment in death. One would be rewarded with heaven, purged by purgatory, or punished in hell. The righteous God will administer reward or punishment on the day of judgment.

The methods of meditation were developed in the Art of Dying. Texts were circulated in the Middle Ages, prescribing guidelines on how to die. The Medieval Art of Dying was an attempt to conceptualize stages of dying in the following order: (1) to pray; (2) seek forgiveness; (3) weep and repent; (4) commend one's soul to God; and (5) give up one's spirit willingly (Helgeland 1984-1985, 155). Normally, dying involved a long, slow process, preceded by premonitions; and witnessed as a public act. If possible, the dying person would face the east, having the arms crossed on the chest. In that position one would receive the sacraments of the Church.

Beginning in the twelfth century, Medieval society underwent a long-term trend of destabilization and disintegration. Some of the causes were poor harvests, economic recession, malnutrition, and chronic overpopulation. These trends were accelerated, further, by the great Bubonic Plague, which swept over Europe between 1348-1350 and destroyed about one quarter of the population. The plague created a vast obsession with death that focused mainly on the body and the processes of decomposition and decay. By 1376 in France the term "macabre" appeared, and it designated the images of the skull, bones, and dried out, emaciated skeletons (Boase 1972, 104).

In the late fourteenth century, the corpse was displayed in an advanced state of decay on transi tombs, the practice lasting until 1600. The term "transi" came from the Latin verb *transire*, meaning "to cross" (*ire*) "over" (*trans*). On these tombs the corpse was viewed publically in its emaciated state, which evoked the feeling of the agony of dying. After burial, a visible effigy of the corpse, sculpted in its skeletal and agonal traits, was made and also displayed publically. On the German transi tombs, in particular, the emaciated corpse was adorned with frogs and worms, or toads and snakes. Typically, frogs were placed on the eyes, mouth, and genitals, and worms encircled the arms and legs.

As a substitute for the bridge, the transi tombs reduced the cross-over motif of dying to anxiety, humiliation, and agony. However, these tombs were restricted to the wealthy, powerful nobility, and royalty, hereby lowered to the level of food for worms and frogs. The intent of the open and public funeral display was to subdue pride, to show that death humiliated the formerly wealthy and powerful, and to undercut worldly glory by the great equalizer of death (Cohen 1973, 12-21). Since frogs and worms were most consistently placed on German tombs, this raises the possibility of a unique interpretation of death. In Revelation 16:13 frogs are "foul spirits" or evil creatures that come "from the mouth of the dragon." In Sirach 10:11 worms mean repentance and frogs sin. These biblical motifs suggest a struggle against evil in death, and they anticipate the same motif in the theology of Martin Luther.

The transi tomb projected imagery of decomposition and decay at the same time that society was disintegrating and displaying primal layers of matter. This trend was represented by the Dance of Death, in which various members of society danced in the roles of naked, rotting, and sexless skeletons. Since participants represented different social classes and they danced as one, the Dance of Death foreshadowed the end of the Medieval hierarchy and the rise of modern notions of equality. As the great equalizer, death waited within one's body to break out and dance.

Underlying these macabre images and practices was a profound psychological disposition. The dying had a passionate attachment to life, a love of things, which turned into a sorrow over their loss (Ariès 1980, 130). To reinforce these material bonds, the devil would bring money with which to tempt the dying. Having to leave all things behind meant that one had failed and, therefore, had become identified with the skeleton as one's ego-ideal. One's skeletal self-image appeared before the onset of sickness and death. Out of this situation comes a philosophy of the object and a psychology of collecting. Because death cuts the living off from collecting things, the need for acquisition remains unsatisfied. Clinging vainly to material things is a form of depression, and in an extreme degree, threatens contact-disintegration, manifesting a sense of being stuck and the illusion of security (Szondi 1980, 256).

These depressive symptoms were the consequences of the disintegration of the bridge symbol.

VI. LUTHER'S RECOVERY OF JOY

Just as the early Middle Ages began with monastic reforms, so in the same way did they end. The order of Augustinian Hermits, founded in 1256, sought reforms in the Roman Catholic Church by restoring strict asceticism, thereby undermining the wealthy and powerful hierarchy and promoting equality among the bishops and priests. Of these monks, Martin Luther was more concerned with the purity of doctrine rather than social change.

Luther decided to enter the monastery on July 2, 1505, when caught in a torrential thunderstorm and thrown to the ground by a bolt of lightning. Shocked by the threat of sudden death, he vowed to become a monk by calling out to St. Ann, patron saint of coal miners. He had descended from a lineage of coal miners through his father Hans and he shared their terror of sudden death by a collapse of the mines.

Within the monastery Luther was taught that one could exist before God by striving for perfection through asceticism, but increasingly he was tormented by anxiety and a sense of unworthiness. He feared rejection by a merciless God. His feeling of unworthiness came, partly from his personal struggle for certainty of faith, and partly from the terror of the age. Fear of an impending end of the world was heightened by Muslim conquests in the Middle East and by recurrent afflictions of the plague. Luther trembled before these onslaughts, believing that they were masks for the devil but fearing that they were signs of the wrath of God. Luther felt the overwhelming spectre of Satan, whom he knew as a radical demonic force that erupts when one seeks the mercy of God.

Confronting the wrath of God exemplifies the fundamental, non-rational dimension of Luther's theology. Luther felt so unworthy before the wrath of God that he wanted to flee. Consequently, he would never fully synthesize the wrath and the love of God in his theology (Miller 1970, 287). Both the wrath and the love interact in an unresolved, dialectical tension; for they reflect the hiddenness of God, the inexhaustible dimension of the "absent God." The traditional dogmatic conception of divine omnipotence was obscured by mystery for Luther, because he believed that attempting to understand it brought neither comprehension nor solace.

In the course of his biblical studies, Luther challenged the Medieval doctrine of the justice of God. With his personal sense of unworthiness, he thought he would not receive righteousness on the day of judgment. His spiritual breakthrough occurred however, when he discovered that, though he be unworthy, Christ is righteous. As stated in Romans 1:17, the righteousness of God has already been disclosed in the crucified Christ. It need only be taken in faith, which means, essentially, trust. Trust in the free gift of grace is the sole content of the gospel.

Despite his crucial discovery, Luther's struggles did not cease. As interpreted by Heiko Oberman, the devil is enraged by the proclamation of the gospel, and he tries to suppress it (1992, 155). For Luther the furious rage of Satan haunts the world and effects the faithful through seizures of temptation. Temptation is a shock of fear that one has been forsaken by God. The shock awakens doubt and drives one to despair. The dilemma is that one strives to save oneself; but this attempt becomes a compulsion that never succeeds in grasping the grace of God. Subjectivity is the obstacle, and the devil is its master.

Receiving the grace of God brings a momentary release from fear, guilt, and unworthiness, and it is experienced as a joyful exchange. In his description of grace Luther captures the biblical meaning of joy, as explained in chapter seven. Grace makes a radiant being, because the will, which is powerless to save itself, is overturned and taken into the mercy of God. With a radiant and loving will, fear and hatred are temporarily conquered.

From this view of the grace of God, Luther developed his theology of death. In **Lectures on Romans** (LW 25, 310) he says that there are two kinds of death (Rom. 6:3). One is temporal, and the other is spiritual. Temporal death is the natural separation of body and soul and seems to be like rest or sleep. Eternal death is a two fold spiritual event. On the one hand, a good spiritual death is a separation of the body from sin and a joining of it with the living God. Death, originally introduced by the devil, is removed through Christ. On the other hand, the bad kind of spiritual death is that of the damned, in which sin and the sinner live eternally. In either case, spiritual death happens only once (Rom. 6:10).

Luther was concerned only with spiritual and not with natural death (Meinhold 1980, 158). Specifically, a good spiritual death absolves the body of its fallenness and creates a new, eternal life under perfect and absolute conditions. As the early Christians knew, it inflicted the death of death. One will never return to life but will remain a cadaver to the world. Since everyone cannot die to the world, baptism is available for the mortification of the flesh. In baptism one dies with Christ and lives toward a good spiritual death.

Because death is essentially a spiritual crisis, how one dies reveals the nature of one's faith. When expounding Romans 6:4, Luther delineates three types of dying. The first consists of the person, who refuses to die and who curses Christ in action and feeling. The second endures dying with great difficulty, groaning, suffering, and finally surrendering in patience. Third, Luther recognizes those who, like Jesus himself, die in joy. Jesus' abject cry of abandonment on the cross was a heroic act of courage and rejoicing.

Luther expanded these insights in "A Sermon on Preparing to Die, 1519" (LW, 42). He says that death is the beginning of a straight and narrow path, which one should walk in joy. Just as the anguish of labor facilitates the birth of a baby, so does sorrow give way to death in joy. Facing death, one may take the sacraments in freedom and joy; for they provide the virtues of strength and power. Sin, death, and hell have no virtue.

Despite the promise of new life, impending death still raises the spectre of the devil. Satan forces humankind to contemplate the horrible images of death and to fear them. The devil cultivates attachments to life, the body, and things, which arouse the wrath of God. The hope of the dying is to meditate on the crucified Christ, whose image alone signifies the revealed love of God. Luther has only signs in his theology and no symbols (Miller 1970, 281). Symbols point beyond themselves, but since the ultimate nature of God is hidden in mystery, symbols provide no meaning. Instead, events are signs that signify, in a clear, unequivocal manner, acts of either God or the devil. In the crucifixion of Jesus the sign of God's love discloses a three fold intentionality: life against death, grace against sin, and heaven against damnation. Reading this sign means that one need not be terrified by death but may give thanks to God in joy.

In a state of radiant being one is elected. Radiant being grounds the affirmation of single predestination, namely, that one has been led into the state of grace by the love and mercy of God. Since the Bible makes the virtue of joy normative, dreams and visions of the night are not needed (Hab. 2:3-4). In his "Table Talk," Luther says that

Gregory, being in the nighttime deceived by a vision, taught something of purgatory, whereas God openly commanded that we should search out and inquire nothing of spirits, but that of Moses and the prophets.

Therefore we must not admit Gregory's opinion on this point; the day of the Lord will show and declare the same, when it will be revealed by fire (Kerr 1943, 243).

Luther refers, of course, to the **Dialogues** of Gregory the Great, but his opinion has been properly disputed on historical and theological grounds. The **Dialogues** are pastorally oriented, and they give no clear evidence of the soul undergoing punishment, as the doctrine of purgatory maintains (Gatch 1969, 113). The purgatory doctrine appeared between 1175-1180, long after Gregory, and only became popular by the end of the thirteenth century (Le Goff 1984, 157, 180, 289). Purgatory was an extension of the sacrament of penance. One would confess one's venial sins before dying and then do penance for them during a specific period of time after death.

Luther appealed to the eschatological fire as the agent of judgment at the end of the world, and he regarded radiant being in the face of death as an anticipation of the cleansing fire. Consequently, he rejected purgatory, dreams, and visions as means of revelation. In **Lectures on Genesis** Luther admits that he has made a pact with God not to receive either dreams or visions (LW. 6, 329). He neither trusts nor seeks dreams and visions, because they can be distorted by the devil. Rather he is content with the biblical text which teaches all things necessary for salvation.

Nevertheless, Luther acknowledges that the Bible speaks of dreams and visions from the age of the fathers to that of the prophets. He notes that the Bible approves of dreams and visions (Numb. 12:6-8; Joel 2:28) and yet disapproves of them (Deut. 13:3; Eccles. 5:7). In order to distinguish between these two perspectives Luther recommends the analogy of faith. Only dreams and visions sent by God are fulfilled in the faith, and fulfillment is determined by two signs: (1) God himself originates them; and (2) he alone provides interpretation and execution. Otherwise, dreams and visions come from the devil, and these are ambiguous and illusory.

The devil can even prophesy through dreams and visions, because he knows some invisible causes and sees ahead to events about 20 or 30 years from now. Consequently, dream interpretation must belong to God, who alone knows all invisible causes. Luther rejects divination, as practiced in Greco-Roman antiquity; for it presumes an independent order of fate outside the will of God. Instead of positing a chain of causes, God allows events to be contingencies that encourage faith, hope, and love.

With his rejection of dreams and visions, it follows that Luther would have no use for the bridge symbol. The symbolism of the bridge presupposes a union of psychic antitheses, which is not possible in Luther's theology. However, he comes close to a bridge equivalent in his exposition of Jacob's ladder in Genesis 28:12-14 (LW. 5). God is on top of the ladder and speaking. On the ladder angels are ascending and descending as spirits and as fire. The ladder signifies the Incarnation, the union of God the Father and God the Son. Only in the crucified Christ do opposites converge, but the unity takes place in the mystery and brutality of Jesus' death. Through the weakness of the dying Jesus, God descends to be like a human being. This offends Satan who wants to ascend and be like God. The devil hates Jacob's ladder.

While Luther withholds a theological reason for dreams and visions, he admits that they may disclose some personal condition. For example, on May 29, 1530 he learned of his father's death and retreated into solitude, grieving deeply, and reading the Psalms. He was so close to his father that

> two nights earlier he had dreamt that he had lost a large tooth, so large that his amazement would not cease. On the Sunday after that his father was dead. At the time a dream of this kind was popularly believed to be an omen of the imminent death of a relative (Oberman 1992, 311).

Just three years earlier, at the beginning of 1527, Luther suffered a seizure of tightness in the throat, a rush of blood to the heart, feeling of cardiac oppression, and painful buzzing in the ears. Combining these symptoms with his well-known fear and trembling, rage and melancholy, Luther appears to be a paroxysmal personality, one subject to the attack syndrome. On July 6, 1527, he suffered a violent circulatory disturbance, followed by depression. He recovered from this illness and lived until 1546.

In February of that year Luther travelled from his home in Wittenberg to Eisleben in order to negotiate a dispute between two parties. While there, he had a premonition of his death and said: "When I get home to Wittenberg again, I will lie down in my coffin and give the worms a fat doctor to feast on" (Cited in Oberman 1992, 5). Luther's remark reflected his knowledge of the Medieval death culture, but in his theology he reversed the meaning of the *Memento Mori*. For Luther the task is not to meditate on death in the midst of life; rather it is to contemplate life in joy.

CONCLUSION:
A THEOLOGY OF DEATH

I. THE ABSENT GOD

Examination of Luther's theology has exposed Jung's critique of Medieval Christianity to be premature. As a Medieval man, Luther had a vision of radical evil in his conception of the Devil as the furious enemy of the Gospel. Although Jung would ground good and evil, life and death in the unconscious, Luther consigned their origins to the unrevealed dimension of God. Out of the absent God came judgment and wrath, which are resolved by the revelation of love and mercy through the death of Jesus. The crucifixion conquered death as the instrument of the Devil.

Luther's doctrine of the absent God envisages an ultimate and irrational mystery in the place of a rational and harmonious universe grounded in the divine mind. His notion of the absent God is also fruitful for a constructive theology of death, as condensed into three governing concepts:

(1) Events of human existence, including death, are contingencies that prepare humankind for God's love and forgiveness. Events are not necessitated by a rational harmonious causality informed by a universal natural law. As contingencies, events betray a spontaneous, seemingly chance-like character and mystery. Luther's rejection of a rational causality comes out of his critique of divination, wherein the Devil foresees future occurrences.

Since events are not strictly determined, death strikes as an unexpected threat, a shock. The fear of sudden death haunted Luther all of his life, and, consequently, he could not make it an object of contemplation. Such a fear implies that death intrudes upon human experience and reverses what is. The contingency of death means that injustice is a primary fact and that it requires justification.

(2) Luther's reversal of Medieval death culture excludes any idea of the stages of dying from a theology of death. Death is neither a natural process nor an object of control. Death is a shock event that readies a natural set of defenses and instinctual drives. Images of dying are useful only in so far as they promote a resolution of suffering. Therefore, so-called stages of dying belong to theodicy.

(3) Revelation of divine grace resolves unjust suffering, and it occurs in a state of joy. Joy comes from surrendering to the will to God. The capacity for surrender is in itself a gift of grace, freely bestowed in the stark cruelty of death. With joy one does not conquer death but participates in the divine love. Such participation creates a radiant being, who bears a total willingness to die. As in the Bible, joy is a function of the will.

Although these three principles be acknowledged, one aspect of Luther's theology needs to be reconstructed. Luther had no theory of symbolism. Instead events are signs, signifying either actions of God or the Devil. The only image Luther admitted was that of the crucified Christ, as the sign of God's love amid death. The omission of symbolism corresponds to his neglect of dreams and visions and his preference for the Scripture as the sole source of religious knowledge. However, Luther conceded that dreams and visions play a pivotal role in biblical history. This admission raises a fundamental dilemma. Dreams and visions are not instruments of revelation, but they belong to the Bible. Hence, dreams and visions cannot be excluded entirely from theology. Clinical experience shows that dreams and visions come to the dying and the bereaved; and this fact restricts them to a psychology of terminal illness and grief work. Our study has demonstrated that dreams and visions facilitate the acceptance of death and the completion of grief work.

Luther's rejection of symbolism followed from his critique of Gregory the Great, and this logically includes Gregory's use of the bridge symbol. In his Genesis commentary Luther interprets Jacob's ladder as a bridge equivalent and as a sign of the Incarnation. For Luther only the crucifixion of Jesus "bridges" life and death, good and evil, strength and weakness. Thus, Luther's theology of death severely narrows the bridge motif but does not eliminate it altogether.

These dilemmas may be resolved by reinstating symbolism into a theology of death. Symbolism is basic to depth psychology and to the history of religions. A symbol combines two principles or dimensions into one and establishes participation between the self and metaphysical reality. A symbol originates from the unconscious and functions as a bridge, spanning image and meaning, foreground and a hidden, transcendent reality (Reimbold 1972, 77). Its validity depends upon whether the bearer sustains a genuine participation with reality. Should participation be lost, then the symbol would disintegrate.

The bridge is a symbol that has become, after Gregory the Great, the normative conception of selfhood in Western civilization. Since the time of Luther, however, the bridge symbol has been viewed in relation to the Roman Catholic papacy. Luther challenged the abuse of Roman power and, thereby, called into question the papal claim to be the exclusive bridge between the divine and the human. While Luther's critique has been essentially accepted, even by Roman Catholicism, it should not obscure the epochal role of the Popes as psychological bridge-builders in the ancient world.

Nevertheless, it is appropriate to wrest the bridge symbol from a specific ecclesiastical structure and to view it in the context of the world religions. Szondi has achieved a fundamental insight into the bridge as a symbol of the participatory self. His vision of the distant shore, as a motif of transcendent reality, coheres with the same conclusion in the work of Frederic Myers. Myers conceived of the distant shore as a symbol of the ecstasy of the supraliminal consciousness. It is the same ecstasy as that of the dreams and visions of death.

The bridge symbol exists in the major world religions, either in a Creation Narrative or eschatology. As a manifestation of the "cross-over" archetype, the bridge is an appropriate symbol for the end of the world. To cross over the bridge to the distant shore means, psychologically, to unify psychic antitheses and to actualize a participatory selfhood. However, as Medieval Christianity demonstrates, the bridge can collapse and give way to depression and despair. So while archaic and enduring, the bridge symbol does not stand as a permanent principle in the evolving universe. It is vulnerable to the primeval shock of death and to the transitoriness of life, as is every symbol. Symbols too come into being and pass away.

II. PRIMORDIAL FREEDOM AND THE FIRE

Going beyond Luther with a theory of symbolism requires a further reconsideration of historical influences. In the seventeenth century the Lutheran mystic, Jacob Boehme, wrestled with the issue of freedom and produced two fundamental contributions to a theology of death. First, he conceived of the absent God as a metaphysical realm in and beyond the physical universe. The absent God became the absolute and primordial realm and was expressed by the German term *Ungrund*. Boehme has made the *Ungrund* a famous idea that has exerted considerable influence upon modern German thought. In his definitive study of Boehme Alexandre Koyré has shown convincingly that *Ungrund* means the total absence of determination, cause, foundation, and reason and that it is properly translated as "absolute" (1968, 280-281).

The second contribution, acknowledged by Koyré, was Boehme's replacing the symbolism of light with that of fire (284, 361-364). Fire symbolizes the primal rhythm of life, and it provides an analogy for the nature of God. Fire remains one, while its internal elements fuse with one another into flaming, radiant energy. Light is not primary but derives from fire. Fire also symbolizes spirit, which is a force and an energy source of nature. To illustrate Koyré quotes from Boehme's **Psychologica Vera** (I, 62):

> Then if there were no fire, there would be no light and also no spirit; and if there were no spirit, so the fire would be extinguished, smothered; and were there darkness and were there one without the other, then nothing; thus both belong together and each participates in the other (fn. 2, 284).

Since fire needs fuel to burn, the fuel is the desire to emerge from the nothingness and to create something. The desire is an incomprehensible will as well as spirit. In Boehme's writing the adjective "incomprehensible" (*ungründige*) is related to the "absolute" (*Ungrund*). Thus, the absolute is an incomprehensible will to create.

Through the symbol of the fire Boehme envisaged the primordial nature of God to be freedom. Freedom is the impulse to become something, to create. He writes in **Six Theosophic Points** that

...the essence of the Deity is everywhere in the deep of the unground [*Ungrund*],...as a wheel or eye, first principle stands in magical quality, and its centre is fire, which cannot subsist without substance; therefore its hunger and desire is after substance (1958, 11-12).

Curiously, Boehme describes the absolute, as though it were a dynamic force rather than a realm without determination. Despite Boehme's considerable vagueness in terminology, he laid down a fundamental insight that has been clarified by Nicolas Berdyaev, "that before being and deeper than being lies the *Ungrund*, the bottomless abyss, irrational mystery, primordial freedom, which is not derivable from being" (1952, 105). Berdyaev correctly states Boehme's intuition of the primacy of freedom as nonbeing over against being. This overturns the ontology of St. Augustine, according to whom God is Being-itself and nonbeing is derived from being.

Even though Berdyaev interprets Boehme correctly, he too confuses terms. Berdyaev's phrase "bottomless abyss" is not an exact rendering of the *Ungrund* but is more consistent with the German *Abgrund*. The conception of the divine abyss actually reenacts the thought of Johannes Tauler, in whose brief writings the idea of the divine "abyss of love" (*Der Abgrund der Liebe*) appears (1961, 71). Tauler was a late Medieval mystic, whose mystical vision of God helped Luther make his Reformation breakthrough (Miller 1970, 261-262). Thus, for Luther and Boehme from the "bottomless abyss" of the absent God the fire of divine love flares up in the darkness of death.

Berdyaev goes on to say that being is "congealed freedom;" it is a "fire which has been smothered and has cooled; but freedom at its fountain head is fiery. This cooling of the fire, this coagulation of freedom is in fact objectification" (111). Berdyaev's interpretation of the fire symbol has far-reaching implications for cosmology and psychiatry as they bear upon a theology of death.

First, it anticipates the idea of the supernova in astronomy. A supernova is the terminal phase of a giant star. When a star begins to die, it contracts into itself because its depleted fuel cannot resist the force of gravity. The star then explodes, blasting energy and matter that turn into the elements of the universe, into calcium, iron, oxygen, and so forth. The fiery heat of the supernova is so great that light radiates in the universe through long wave-lengths. The vibrating, radiant light from a dying star may be seen telescopically thousands of light-years away.

Frederic Myers considered the death of a star as an exact analogy for the veridical afterimage of death. The new concept of the supernova updates Myers' analogy. Further, the analogy of the supernova illumines a fundamental characteristic of shock death, as confirmed by death-bed visions and NDEs, namely, acceleration of thought. Thus, in the human terminal phase thought accelerates to a peak of luminous intensity, where it implodes in death and ecstasy, releasing the explosive afterimage. Just as a dying star contracts, so does the person. The human being contracts to the point of total stillness, where space, time, and physical being cease.

Second, Boehme's fire symbolism anticipates aspects of psychiatry, as represented particularly by Szondi. In this book on therapy Szondi takes up the issue of the *Ungrund* and defines it correctly as the realm of absolute indifference, which lacks all antitheses (1963, 34). The *Ungrund* cannot be posited directly, he says; it can only be affirmed indirectly by negation. Szondi also contends that the notion of the *Ungrund* conforms to the theory of the unconscious; for out of the unconscious arises a "drive of all impulses and representations to emerge into consciousness, to transcend" (35). The capacity to emerge from the unconscious belongs to the psyche, which is the fundamental drive toward freedom, specifically, the drive toward social and metaphysical participation. However, Szondi confuses terms as well; for in discussing the *Ungrund*, he shifts to *Urgrund*, which Koyré defines as the "absolute as ground and as first cause of things" (1968, 281). The notion of *Urgrund* implies an active power in the sense of a dynamic unconscious, a primal force, as posited particularly by Freud.

Despite the semantic confusion, a basic coherence exists. Szondi's description of psyche as a drive toward freedom coincides with our definition of mind as act, in chapter six. Acts of mind constitute a process, in which consciousness and unconsciousness function as phases. Mental acts cannot be located precisely in physical entities or spatio-temporal forms. In the face of death they accelerate to a peak of luminous intensity, which is also the drive of the psyche for freedom and participatory being.

Clinically, acceleration of thought occurs in paroxysmal-epileptiform phenomena. Epilepsy conceals an unconscious depth, which even eludes neurology. The depth dimension of epilepsy is expressed through the seizure, both as a defense against the impact of death and as a search for meaning and value, atonement and wholeness. Atonement and wholeness are sought through symbolism, specifically, through motifs of ascent and descent, height and depth, vortex and wave, also through the elements of air, earth, water, and fire. Of the elemental symbols, fire has priority, because its leaping, flaring nature expresses the volcanic convulsions of epilepsy and the refinement of the aura, as Dostoevsky knew.

Thus, in conclusion, the symbolism of fire, as exemplified in the supernova and epileptic seizure, converges with a theology of death. In the darkness of death the psyche accelerates in a "fiery" epileptiform process to a peak of luminous intensity, defending against death in shock suffering and driving to an exalted state of freedom. The upsurge of the psyche reenacts the Creation, when in the beginning the Creative fire flared up from the dark primeval abyss of God, swept across the waters of chaos, and brought forth light (Gen. 1:2-3). The psychic drive for freedom in death also anticipates the eschatological fire, which Luther foresaw as a sign of judgment and redemption of the end of the world. The eschatological fire burns with the radiance of the crucifixion afterimage.

III. DEATH AS CONTINGENCY

In this and the next two sections the governing guidelines of a theology of death are explored through three personal situations. First, Luther's haunting sense of the contingency of death and the absent God culminated in the theology and experience of Paul Tillich. Tillich's biographer reports that he struggled against death his entire life (Pauck 1976, 1-2). For Tillich death would never be a noble friend or personal fulfillment but, rather, the stranger. Death is the realm of total, incomprehensible darkness.

Tillich's life-long dread of death was shaped by two traumas. One was the death of his mother, when he was 17 years old. He represses the fact of her death and projected his love for her on "to the sea and to the sun" (15). Thereafter, Tillich cultivated an attraction to the dark, tragic side of nature, especially symbolized by the heavy waves of the ocean crashing against a rocky shore at twilight.

The other trauma was his service as an army chaplain in World War I. Tillich understood the war to be the destruction of an entire world order, the collapse of civilization into chaos. Once, during heavy combat, he wrote to a friend:

> I have constantly the most immediate and very strong feeling that I am no longer alive. Therefore I don't take life seriously, to find someone, to become joyful, to recognize God, all these things are things of life. But life is not dependable ground. It isn't only that I might die any day, but rather that everyone dies, *really* dies, you too....(51)

The shock of total death exposed the dark nothingness, the *Ungrund* of the absent God. In the trenches Tillich realized that a rational conception of a personal theism no longer made sense. The love of God could not be reconciled with "the sound of exploding shells, of weeping at open graves, of the sighs of the sick, of the moaning of the dying" (49). When in a French forest, however, Tillich read Friedrich Nietzsche's **Thus Spoke Zarathustra** and became inspired by the author's ecstatic affirmation of life.

The biographer does not state Nietzsche's exact impact on Tillich, but a clue appears in his sermon on "The Depth of Existence," which is based on two biblical texts (Tillich 1948, 52-53). From Psalm 130:1 he takes the Hebrew image of Sheol and redefines it as depth; and with I Corinthians 2:10 he makes depth a spiritual dimension. Depth is "infinite and inexhaustible," and it is God. Toward the end of the sermon Tillich says that the way into depth leads to joy:

> ...joy is deeper than suffering. It is ultimate. Let me express this in the words of a man who, in passionate striving for the depth, was caught by destructive forces and did not know the word to conquer them. Friedrich Nietzsche writes: "The world is deep, and deeper than the day could read. Deep is its woe. Joy deeper still than grief can be. Woe says: Hence, go! But joys want all eternity, want deep, profound eternity" (63).

This passage is a quotation of Zarathustra's "Midnight Song," after which Tillich states: "The moment in which we reach the last depth of our lives is the moment in which we can experience the joy that has eternity within...."

In subsequent sermons Tillich explored the meaning of joy as basic to a theology of death. Joy is neither pleasure nor happiness; for joy can be attained in their opposites, in pain and unhappiness (Tillich 1955, 145, 149). The search for pleasure evades pain but cannot produce joy. Rather, joy correlates with sorrow, which expresses death, grief, and the transitoriness of life. Only joy has the ability to embrace sorrow and, consequently, to experience the eternal.

This theme appeared in Tillich's Easter sermon of 1964, which I heard him deliver at a university chapel in Massachusetts. With only 18 months to live, Tillich declared that in the crucifixion of Jesus "death is taken into life, the pain of having to come to [an] end is taken into the joy of being here and now" (1964, 8). In joy the end changes; it comes here and now, not after death:

> If death is accepted by us already, we do not need to wait for it, be it near or far, be it with fear or with contempt. We know what it is because we have accepted it in all its darkness and tragedy. We know that it is the confirmation that we are creatures and that our end belongs to us. We know that life cannot be prolonged, neither in this nor in some imagined future existence.

Then in a dramatic and poignant moment, he concluded his sermon with a prayer: "Give me strength to take my death into my life! Amen."

Tillich's own end came in October, 1965, when he suffered a heart attack and began to die. His dying process was witnessed by his wife Hannah (H. Tillich 1973, 220-225). Speaking to her from his hospital bed, he said: "I live mostly in dreams now. Everything is slipping away under my feet...in these hours of the emptiness of time." He saw a river of depleted, empty time, going on and on, in night and horror, while being "delivered to the vast ocean of impenetrable depth." His doctors interpreted these images as projections of his own anxiety, but Tillich insisted that they were real.

On the first evening of his hospitalization, he had this dream:

> I awoke and found myself in a situation which was very uncanny. One of my thoughts was, I have died. I see a man who is very interesting and who has in a certain way very sympathetic features. He says to me, "You know what

happened?" Then "You know what happened to Hannah?" I
asked, "Did she die?" He answers, "Yes. Somebody perished
on a trip." My first thought, "Is it Rene?" [Tillich's son]
"Yes"....

The other man in the dream is Tillich's own background self that
expresses an unconscious aggression of his death onto family members.
The dream reveals his ambivalence about death, which the earlier images
had portrayed as a dark, bottomless abyss of nothingness.

On the next day, Tillich remembered friends who had died during the
previous decade and in World War I. These recollections were a *deja
vu* or life review: "One sees the enormous problems of the bodies and
how refined the body is when it is taken as an organism [in the hospital],
and how brutal it is when it is all cut into pieces [by cannons]."

Hannah encouraged her husband to let all these images float away.
"Go after the clear light," she said, "the clear light will guide you, not
any self-centered immortality." She urged him to "realize the voidness."
He then began to lose "all differentiation between himself and others....
No longer was there any distinction between friend or foe. There was
no otherness." He confessed his earlier behavior, as it had effected their
marriage, and received forgiveness from Hannah. Finally, realizing his
total wholeness and awareness, she grasped his hand, then suddenly, he
let go; "his body pranced as if in ecstasy...he fell back, his mouth was
open...."

Tillich's death had occurred through ecstatic phases of dreaming,
recollection, and the intellectual aura of emptiness. This paroxysmal-
epileptiform death expressed mainly the elemental symbols of water and
the refined light of fire. Psychoanalytically, his slipping into the
inexhaustible ocean depth was a return to his mother.

IV. DEATH AS INJUSTICE

Peter Noll was a Swiss law professor and judge, who developed a
malignant tumor on his kidney, partially covering the urethra. His
physicians told him that surgery could be performed successfully but that
it would leave him impotent. Noll feared that if he were to undergo
surgery, he would also lose his independence. Without shock, anger, or
despair, Noll considered the tumor to be a case of bad luck. However,

since he had been divorced, he realized that his cancer was a direct result of the separation.

Noll rejected surgery; for he believed the will to live must prevail against the indignity of medical dependence. After making this decision, he decided to keep a diary, while even knowing that his writing would not change anything. The diary narrates ideas, feelings, and events in his life from December 28, 1981 to September 30, 1982. He died on October 9, 1982, and his diary was published later under the title **In the Face of Death** (Noll 1990). At the time of his death Noll was 56 years old.

He admits in surprise that he feels freer, more aware, and more intense, as he writes with knowledge of the brevity of life. Ironically, he thinks that books written by terminal cancer patients express helplessness and embarrassment. Cancer books mirror an affluent society, where complaints against death are narcissistic and filled with self-pity (213).

He was the son of a Swiss Reformed pastor and well-versed in theology. Having chosen to confront death directly, he identified with Jesus, as one who died individually and for all those who died unjustly:

> Jesus did accept His own death willingly as full reality and fought it through to the end—i.e., His vision of the kingdom of God and paradise in no way diminishes death's terror. Thus, nowhere in the Bible are dying and death trivialized. Jesus wanted at first that the cup pass from Him; at the end he thought that God had forsaken Him.
>
> ...He wanted to accept dying and death in all its seriousness, without a glance to the "compensations" of paradise. The idea that the soul leaps out of the body and escapes into beautiful fields of eternity was absolutely foreign to Him (29-30).

That Jesus sought no compensation could be taken as a criticism of Jungian psychology, according to which the unconscious projects a mythic afterlife to offset the brutality of death. Noll declares that even with the compensation of immortality, his tumor and his death remain. Guided only by the image of the crucified Christ, he becomes more calm and patient. He even has no dreams or visions.

From the beginning of his illness, Noll planned his funeral, feeling both sorrow and joy but no despair. He confided that the reality of death should be cultivated as a way to understand freedom. One's own freedom and conscience reveal God's freedom (149). Just as death relativizes life, so does the divine freedom relativize human events. Events become contingencies.

In April, 1982 Noll travelled to Egypt, where he acquired a viral infection and became seriously ill. Red drops of blood flowed in his urine. He had shortness of breath, cold sweating, nausea, and dizziness. Returning home to Zürich, he knew that he had been close to death. He realized then that "death assumes a higher quality when it is more conscious. The only question is whether in dying this activity of consciousness is still possible, and for how long" (155).

Interwoven throughout the diary are incisive analyses of the problems of justice, power, and law. Even though human consciousness resists change, he argues, society should organize itself to achieve meaningful transformation. Yet organizations yield to dominance hierarchies, whose intolerance is a driving force of evil. Hence, the human task is to make law right and just, since social order is a function of law and not of power. The problem of power arises because of the fundamental condition of injustice inherent in the human condition.

As Noll laments injustice, he confesses the unfairness of dying (187). Suddenly, it becomes apparent to the reader that Noll believes his own death is unfair, and that this unfairness reveals the basic injustice of existence. Thus, his argument that law is a critique of power implies that law is also a critique of death. Further, the preservation of injustice in the structures of social organizations parallels the abnormal growth of the cancer tumor. Hence, the political task of reversing injustice complements the need to find a justification for the unfairness of death.

To discharge his anger against injustice Noll reads the prophet Isaiah, "whose blazing sword of fire is what it took to hold his own against the powers of his day" (135). He admires Isaiah for keeping conscience and freedom in the name of God, but he concedes that the prophets are all gone. Instead the clergy preach sterile dichotomies of sin and grace, which only personalize world events and overlook the fact that

the totality of events with all its participants has gone wrong and must be replaced by something new. Hence, with a certain inner logic, prophecy turns to apocalyptic. For Jesus, the end of the world was imminent (167).

Prophecy turns to apocalyptic when "the objective and uncontrollable conditions, the immanent logic of the systems, are even stronger than a majority of well-intentioned people" (168). Not even the rage of the prophet could halt the inexorable fate of events, Noll laments. His vision of the inexorable fate of events parallels the uncontrollable advance of his own cancer. When cancer dominates the body, simple dichotomies of pain and pleasure, loss and happiness collapse, and one lives with masked pain, masked grief, and masked despair.

> Perhaps only through pain...do we become aware that life is mostly toil, interrupted now and then by little oases of meaning. Thus pain would have a metaphysical meaning, by revealing that this world, at least since the existence of man, is dominated by evil and that transcendent good succeeds only occasionally in bringing joy to the individual. Developed logically, this thought means that joy and good deeds are signs from a better world beyond (203-204).

Pain is metaphysical, because it discloses that "eternity abolishes time, space, and causality" (215). Only in an "oasis of meaning" may God be experienced.

Throughout the late summer of 1982, Noll's pain so intensified that he lost all appetite and felt mainly nausea and fatigue. He even gave up morphine, because it was ineffective. Finally, in early October he asked his daughter Rebecca to take care of him. She writes in his diary that on the morning of October 9, she

> was supporting his heavy head with mine, was dabbing the sweat from his face, feeling now and then whether his heart was still beating. Suddenly something startled me, despite total silence and darkness.
>
> Then he began to heave deeply and painfully. I thought to myself, my God, how could you let anybody suffer like this! and almost at the same time, Yes, God does let people suffer. At that moment my father ceased breathing (247).

V. DEATH AS RADIANT SUFFERING

Ben Oyler was diagnosed in May, 1985, when he was only seven years old, as an AIDS patient. The story of his death has been told by his mother Chris (Oyler 1990). He was born a hemophiliac and been given many blood transfusions to supply the missing protein necessary for clotting. Chris estimates that Ben had been exposed to the blood of 48,000 persons, one of whom carried the AIDS virus (31). With hemophilia the mother is the carrier, and her male children have a 50% chance of acquiring the disease. Thus, hemophilia is X-linked recessive, and all three of the Oyler boys suffered it. Chris' brother Scott was born with hemophilia and glaucoma, which made him blind by age eight. Chris had informed Grant, her husband that she might be a carrier, when they became engaged; but he said: "It doesn't matter" (71).

During the early spring of 1985, Ben constantly felt sick to his stomach. He suffered diarrhea and vomiting but, instead of going away, these conditions persisted and brought fatigue as well as weight loss. Ben also acquired a rash and a white coating in the throat, which was a contagious infection. His neck swelled, and he developed a thick, deep cough. The family physician referred Ben to Stanford Children's Hospital, where he received his AIDS diagnosis and given one year to live.

The shock of the diagnosis made Chris numb. She had to struggle with the anguished image of Ben, his increasingly sunken eyes and narrow face. In anger she cried out:

Oh Ben, why did it have to be you?
Why Ben? Why Ben? How many times had I asked myself that question. Of all the innocent victims, Why did Ben have to get AIDS? It was so unfair. What had we done to deserve this? (33, 37, 53)

Throughout the remaining months of 1985, Chris grieved for his deteriorating, skeletal being, his skinny, little legs, wide mouth and emaciated face. Occasionally, her anger would mix with denial, when wishing she could reverse time and go back to before Ben's random but fatal transfusion (53).

His agonizing, cramping pain was diagnosed as pancreatitis, which was treated with pain medication and intubation through the nose and throat to drain off gastric fluids. This, in turn, was followed by a case of the shingles, which caused Chris to become numb again and then derealized.

In contrast, Ben did not exhibit grief-related phases of denial, anger, derealization, or numbness, but instead he expressed symbolic language. After Jessica, a first grade classmate, had died of cancer, he talked about her with his mother:

> "Will Jessica go to heaven?"
> "Yes."
> "Will I see her again someday?"
> "I'm sure you will, Ben."
> There was a long silence. Ben just kept looking down and drawing in the sand.
> "When will that be, Mom?"
> "I don't know, Ben" (59).

Ben's question reflects innate knowledge of his own dying, as projected in the symbol of the heavenly journey. Shortly after, the family arranged for Ben's baptism and, during preparations, he asked: "Are there tacos in heaven?" (66) Still later, when discussing his condition with his maternal grandmother, he expressed his knowledge of death more directly. The grandmother told Chris that "Ben knows he's going to die and he's afraid you and Grant are going to be mad at him...he wanted me to call you" (85).

Along with this realization came a leave-taking ritual, when Ben decided to sell his bike. Chris recalls:

> I think that was the moment I realized how Ben was changing. Things like bicycles and break dancing and school didn't matter so much to Ben any more. His mind, indeed his soul, was working toward something greater.
>
> It was like the stories you hear about people who get an incredible surge of power and energy in an emergency. Power they never knew they had, Ben had that. Deep inside him there was a source that helped him understand and accept and not be afraid (106).

She also explains that Ben had begun to mature shortly after the diagnosis, a fact even observed by the medical staff. Psychoanalysts might attribute Ben's enhancement of power to be infantile omnipotence, but this would be contradicted by Ben's deepening character and feeling. Ben does not regress, but he progresses.

Ironically, as Ben matures psychically, he stops growing physically and begins to lose control. For example, shortly before Christmas Eve, 1985, he walked into a door jamb, fell, and nearly knocked himself unconscious (154). Sometime later, an emergency code sounded in the hospital. Chris ran down the corridor into the room and saw "Ben's little body jerking up and down on the bed, over and over and over again. Never, never, had I seen a body go through such violent movement" (163). Ben had suffered a grand mal epileptic seizure, after which he said with "barely a whisper:"

"Mom, I want to go home."
Ben had to say it twice before I realized what he was saying.
He didn't mean Carmel. He meant really going home. We had
told Ben dying was like going home. And now he was ready
(163-164).

Informed by the doctors that seizures usually occur in pairs, Ben's parents waited for another attack. Meanwhile, they signed papers requesting no extraordinary, life-support treatment for Ben. As expected, Ben had his second grand mal seizure, and it came at 11:00 p.m. on a spring night of 1986.

Grant and I held Ben down and I could feel the convulsions
wrack Ben's body over and over and over again.
For me, it was more terrifying than the first. Not because
the seizure was worse; it was clearly milder. But because this
time Ben was awake when it started. This time he would
remember it happening (190).

Chris had asked the doctors for a neurological explanation of Ben's fall and his two grand mal seizures, but she received none. As discussed in chapter one, neurology cannot fully explain epilepsy, particularly its psychiatric aspects and its relation to death. Only the psychiatric view, as maintained by Szondi, could answer Chris' question. Hence, two epileptic convulsions indicate accelerated affect in defense against Ben's impending death as well as a search for meaning in death, specifically, acceptance through the symbol of the heavenly journey. Ben's fall would derive from a weakened bodily condition and from an unconscious disposition associated with the paroxysmal-epileptiform situation.

After the second seizure, the doctors increased Ben's pain medication. With Ben's slightly slurred speech, Chris feared that he might not be able to communicate clearly.

> "I'm afraid it'll hurt, Mom," he said.
> "We'll get you some different medicine, Ben."
> "I mean when I die, Mom."
> I looked at Ben and my heart stood still.
> There was total acceptance written on his face. No panic. No fear. None of the denial and confusion I felt in my own heart. Just something that said: I knew this was going to happen and I can handle it, I'm ready, but I just need a little help (194).

With each epileptic convulsion, Ben's father Grant suffered two attacks himself. He said: "I just felt this pain go down my arm, and couldn't breathe, and I almost fell over" (184). The doctors diagnosed these as "stress attacks," brought on by the pressure of work, mounting medical bills, family tension, and personal grief. In contrast, I interpret the two episodes as paroxysmal-hysteriform anxiety attacks, caused by his decision to remain psychically detached from Ben's terminal illness. The term stress comes from physics; and it refers to the impact of physical forces upon systems like buildings or bridges. It is unsuited to human beings, who struggle with feelings and crises. The notion of anxiety fits Grant's dilemma, more precisely, because he felt helpless and vulnerable, unable to stay in control. Anxiety expresses the shock of helplessness in the face of death.

It is necessary to interpret his attacks as anxiety-induced in order to understand what happened next. Grant clenched his fist and smashed one of his son's cribs. Smashing the crib is hardly reducible to stress. Instead it is a violent discharge of anger or the Cain tendency in defense against the dread of death. He had been seized by the same pent-up emotion that had unconsciously driven Ben's epileptic seizures. When viewed together, both father and son had released a paroxysmal-epileptiform defense against death.

With Grant's destruction of the crib, Chris resents her husband's failure to cope; so she withdraws from him. Having been closer to Ben, Chris feels that her own anxiety had diminished, particularly after one poignant experience:

> Sometimes we'd go to the beach to watch the waves crash into the shore, or to spot the seals gallivanting about the rocks.
>
> We'd sit there on the sand and recall special times we had spent in the past.
>
> There was a peaceful quality about our times together. The noise was gone now. That noise in my ears that sounded like the hum of a million fluorescent lights.
>
> That hum was the sound of fear. And when I stopped being afraid, it went away. And in its place was a quiet grief. Sad but peaceful (212-213).

Chris has reached a profound sorrow beyond anxiety, because she had surrendered to Ben's dying process. Her sorrow prepared the way for joy, of which the Psalms, Luther, and Tillich have spoken. Chris' depth of feeling was achieved at the ocean, where identification with the undulating rhythm of the waves renewed her. Consciously, going to the ocean signified her need for peace, but unconsciously and archetypally it symbolized descent to the primal origin of life.

Meanwhile, Ben approaches death with enhanced control. He requests that his doctors remove his nasogastric tube, and he signs his will, formally bequeathing his bicycle to his brother Beau. As death grew closer, Grant had to leave Ben's bed. Chris laments: "He could not bear to sit by our son's death-bed. And I could not bear to leave" (225).

Shortly before Ben's death, his brother Aber exclaimed: "There's a little ghost flying around in my room." His grandmother said it was just a bad dream, but Aber insisted: "It was Ben. He came in here and told me that he won't have to hurt anymore 'cause he's got only one more day here. He told me he loved me and he'd miss me a lot" (228-229).

Early the next morning, as Grant sat beside her, Chris said to her dying son: "Ben, do you see a light? A warm and comforting light? Follow it. It's there for you...." Ben felt limp, and she reached for his hand, as though he were falling. She "felt the immense power of the pain he was releasing;" but then her fear vanished, as she was enveloped in a radiant afterimage:

> The room was full of Ben. He was all around us, everywhere. Warm and loving. He was lingering there for a moment to say good-bye. To tell us not to worry, that there wasn't anything to be afraid of, and never was (229-230).

VI. JOY AND RADIANT BEING

Ben Oyler's terminal illness presents a compelling challenge to a theology of death. The suffering of an innocent child subverts the natural order of the world. The child dies before the parents. The child does not grow up, marry, produce children, and transmit genes to the next generation. The child barely lives long enough to deepen psychic antitheses and, thus, to bridge them.

The death of a child poses a potential obstacle to the primary task of grief work, namely, an actual acceptance of the loss. Acceptance is difficult because the child is an extension of the parent. Consequently, the death of a child also means the death of a parent. Hence, Chris Oyler expresses considerable astonishment, when, in the epilogue of her book, she describes her only bereavement dream:

> He was taller than he used to be, grown up, as if he had never been sick. He stood out in the middle of a crowd and I went to him. But, as I opened my arms for his embrace, he stepped back. "Don't you know, Mom?" he whispered. "You can't touch me here" (236).

The dream has the characteristic of a normal bereavement dream, signifying the completion of grief work. The dream also reveals the cessation of contact-bonding between mother and son and the attainment of the son's primal form in death. His mandate for her is that she must withdraw her projections from him.

Psychoanalytically, this dream narrates a transition from the biological mother to mother earth, who destroys the male, since she loves him the most. In an essay on the three fates of Greek mythology Freud argues that the three goddesses of fate represent the three women in the destiny of the male: the mother who bears him, the woman who marries him, and the mother earth, the goddess of death (1958, S.E., XII). Because mother earth takes the man in death, he must endure dying as a cruel necessity of nature.

Jung would also acknowledge the brutality of death but assign it to the ego. The death of the ego is compensated by the unification of the self in the eternal, or unconscious. One attains a primal form in death, which is manifest as joy. Thus, death has been portrayed traditionally as a wedding, Jung contends. "On Greek sarcophagi the joyous element was represented by dancing girls, on Etruscan tombs by banquets. When the pious Cabbalist Rabbi Simon ben Jochai came to die, his friends said that he was celebrating his wedding" (Jung 1961, 314-315).

While the judgments of Freud and Jung are realistic and meaningful, neither fits the suffering death of an eight year old boy. Freud's mythic appeal to mother earth as the loving goddess of death trivializes Chris Oyler's profound and anguished suffering. Jung's image of the wedding expresses the union of psychic antitheses but presumes the entire life cycle to remain intact, conditions obviously unfitting for the limited span of a prepubescent boy.

A more accurate view emerges, when considering that the exact cause of Ben's death was two-fold: hereditary hemophilia which created the need for blood transfusions and the infection by tainted blood from one out of 48,000 donors. The hereditary cause involves a 50% probability ratio, and the infection seems to be a virtual matter of chance. Both factors comprise a contingency, but once the virus has been acquired, the disease process unfolds as an irreversible necessity. Ben Oyler's situation entails a primary contingency and a derivative necessity. The unfolding of a pattern of necessity from a contingent cause constitutes the nature of destiny (Hughes 1992, 165).

Of the depth psychologists studied in this book only Szondi assigns priority to the order of destiny. Destiny expresses the basic human condition, of which terminal illness plays an integral role. Concentrating on destiny does not sanction a determinism or deny freedom. In a lecture delivered in 1954 and published posthumously, Szondi argues that humankind does not come into the world by chance but for responsibility (1954/1989, 55). The human task is to achieve participation in a transcendent, spiritual realm, to which one surrenders one's entire being joyously. The spiritual surrender is a withdrawal of the will, a suspension of the drive to dominate the physical world, wherein the spatio-temporal forms of life mask the anxiety of death.

Metaphysically, the order of destiny presupposes a primal freedom. As with Boehme and Berdyaev, freedom precedes life and being and manifests a dynamic nonbeing. Being takes shape in the three dimensional order of space, time, and causality, the order through which the will achieves material domination as a defense against death. The derivative order of being also projects the basic antitheses of good and evil, consciousness and unconsciousness, sickness and health and so forth. Theologically, primal freedom is expressed in the biblical Creation Narrative, when the divine spirit sweeps across the waters of chaos and produces light from darkness (Gen.1:1-4). Because of the primacy of watery chaos, which is connected to Sheol, darkness has priority in the doctrine of God. The divine darkness precludes arguments as to the positive and rational attributes of God. The theology of death belongs to the tradition of the negative (*apophatic*) theology.

It follows theologically that God does not inflict terminal illness; it just happens. With hereditary causes, the ancestors "send" diseases upon their descendants, not so much as punishment but as a means of preservation. Modern biology teaches that genes seek to reproduce themselves by creating multiple copies and unconscious processes of reciprocal attraction among their bearers. This is as true for the genes of hemophilia as for those of epilepsy. Although not yet confirmed, the same genotropic tendency may belong to the AIDS virus. Yet whether medical causes be fully established or not, the ultimate causality lies in the freedom of being. This fundamental postulate also accords with the conclusion of Frederic Myers, who found no evidence for a determinism underlying death-related psychic events.

Positing the metaphysical primacy of freedom and nonbeing means that death can be neither conquered nor integrated. This perspective deviates from that of Tillich, who struggled against the dread of death, because his inclination was to incorporate nonbeing into being, death into life. His personal view reflected his theological judgment that God is Being-itself and, therefore, that being precedes nonbeing. Tillich maintained the theological ontology of St. Augustine, even as he interpreted the vision of Luther with great intellectual power.

While Augustinian ontology retains integrity, it is difficult to reconcile it clinically with degenerative diseases. The latter threaten chronic, unmanageable pain, leading to disintegration and despair. Peter Noll did not integrate nonbeing into being; for his severe and debilitating pain shattered the spatio-temporal and causal forms of his existence.

Chronic pain has the power to undermine the will, erode mastery, and inflict a total helplessness in the face of the savage, irrational forces of despair. Chronic pain discloses the darkness of the primal abyss and the absent God.

Though nearly broken by pain, Noll affirmed the principle of freedom as ultimate and surrendered to the darkness in praise. The capacity to praise means that one has achieved radiant being, participation in fundamental reality, as illuminated forever by the crucifixion afterimage.

REFERENCES

I. SOURCES IN BIBLICAL STUDIES

Anderson, Gary. 1991. **A Time To Mourn, A Time To Dance.** University Park, PA: Pennsylvania State University Press.

Arndt, William and Gingrich, F.W. 1979. **A Greek-English Lexicon of the New Testament.** 2nd ed. Chicago: University of Chicago Press.

Astour, Micheal. 1980. "The Nether World and its Denizens at Ugarit." **Death in Mesopotamia**, ed. B. Alster. Copenhagen: Akademisk Forlag, 227-238.

Bottero, Jean. 1980. "La Mythologie de la Morten Mesopotamie Ancienne." **Death in Mesopotamia**, ed. B. Alster. Copenhagen: Akademisk Forlag, 25-52.

Finkel, Irving. 1983-1984. "Necromancy in Ancient Mesopotomia." **Archiv für Orientforschung** XXIX, 1-17.

Gardner, John and Maier, John, trans. 1984. **Gilgamesh.** New York: Alfred A. Knopf.

Gray, John. 1961. "Texts From Ras Shamra." **Documents from Old Testament Times**, ed. D.W. Thomas. New York: Harper & Brothers, 116-133.

Grayston, Kenneth. 1952. "The Darkness of the Cosmic Sea." **Theology** LV, 122-127.

Healey, J.F. 1980. "The Sun Deity and The Underworld." **Death in Mesopotamia**, ed. B. Alster. Copenhagen: Akademisk Forlag 239-242.

Jacob, Edmond. 1962. "Death." **Interpreter's Dictionary of the Bible**, 802-804.

Kee, Howard, Young, Franklin, and Froehlich, Karlfried. 1973. **Understanding the New Testament**. 3rd. ed. Englewood Cliffs, NJ: Prentice-Hall.

Kugel, James. 1986. "Topics in the History of the Spirituality of the Psalms." **Jewish Spirituality**, ed. A. Green. New York: Crossroad, 113-144.

Lambert, W.G. ed. 1960. **Babylonian Wisdom Literature**. Oxford: Oxford University Press.

Muffs, Yochanan. 1975. "Joy and Love as Metaphorical Expressions of Willingness and Spontaneity." **Christianity, Judaism and Other Greco-Roman Cults**, ed. J. Neusner. Vol. III. Leiden: E J. Brill, 1-36.

Müller, Hans-Peter, 1978. "Gilgameschs Trauergesang um Enkidu und die Gattung der Totenklage." **Zeitschrift für Assyiologie** 68 (2), 233-250.

Pedersen, Johs. 1926. **Israel: Its Life and Culture**. Vol I. London: Geoffrey Cumberlege.

Perrin, Norman. 1977. **The Resurrection According to Matthew, Mark, and Luke.** Philadelphia: Fortress Press.

Rengstorf, K.H. 1953. **Die Anfänge der Auseinandersetzung zwischen Christusglaube und Asklepiosfrömmigkeit.** Münster: Aschendorff.

Silberman, Lou. 1969. "Death in the Hebrew Bible and Apocalyptic Literature." **Perspectives on Death**, ed. L. Mills. Nashville: Abingdon Press.

Tigay, Jeffrey. 1982. **The Evolution of the Gilgamesh Epic**. Philadelphia: University of Pennsylvania Press.

Tromp, Nicholas. 1969. **Primitive Conceptions of Death and the Nether World in the Old Testament**. Rome: Pontifical Biblical Institute.

Weber,Hans-Reudi. 1979. **The Cross**, trans. E. Jessett. Grand Rapids: Wm. B. Eerdman's Publishing Co.

II. SOURCES IN BIOLOGY

Bereczkei, Tamás. 1992. "Biological Evolution, Genotropism, Psychopathology." **Szondiana** 12(2), 32-52.

Dawkins, Richard. 1976. **The Selfish Gene**. New York: Oxford University Press.

Dobzhansky, Theodosius. 1970. **Genetics of the Evolutionary Process**. New York: Columbia University Press.

Harris, Ann and Super, Maurice. 1987. **Cystic Fibrosis**. New York: Oxford University Press.

Milunsky, Aubrey. 1989. **Choices, Not Chance**. Boston: Little, Brown.

Smith, J. Maynard. 1964. "Group Selection and Kin Selection." **Nature** 201 (March 14), 1145-1147.

III. SOURCES IN DEATH STUDIES

Barrett, William. 1926/1986. **Death-Bed Visions**. Northamptonshire: The Aquarian Press.

Booth, Gotthard. 1979. "Psychobiological Aspects of 'Spontaneous' Regression of Cancer." **Stress and Survival**, ed. C. Garfield. St. Louis: C. V. Mosby.

Brooks, Kakie. 1991. "Near-death Experiences." **The Observer Magazine**. (June 13/ June 19), 3,22.

Cooke, Mary. 1976. "Death With Dignity-Hawaiian Style." **Honolulu Advertiser** (June 24). Sec. C, 1-2.

Coolidge, Frederick and Fish, Cynthia. 1983-1984. "Dreams of the Dying." **Omega** 14(1), 1-7.

Dreifuss-Kattan, Esther. 1990. **Cancer Stories**. Hillsdale, NJ: The Analytic Press.

Gabbard, Glen and Twemlow, Stuart. 1984. **With The Eyes of the Mind**. New York: Praeger.

Garfield, Charles. 1979. "The Dying Patient's Concern with 'Life After Death.'" **Between Life & Death**, ed. R. Kastenbaum. New York: Springer.

Greyson, Bruce. 1985. "A Typology of Near-Death Experiences." **American Journal of Psychiatry** 142(8), 967-969.

Gorer, Geoffrey. 1973. "Death, Grief, and Mourning in Britain." **The Child and His Family**, ed. E. J. Anthony and C. Koupenik. New York: John Wiley.

Heim, Albert. 1892/1972. "The Experience of Dying from Falls," trans. R. Noyes and R. Kletti. **Omega** 3(1), 45-52.

Holck, Frederick. 1978-1979. "Life Revisited: Parallels in Death Experiences." **Omega** 9(1), 1-11.

Hoyt, Michael. 1980-1981. "Clinical Notes Regarding the Experience of 'Presences' in Mourning." **Omega** 11(2), 105-111.

Hufford, David. 1982. **The Terror that Comes in the Night**. Philadelphia: University of Pennsylvania Press.

Hughes, Richard. 1990. "My Father's Death." **Lycoming Quarterly** 6(2), 13-14, 20.

Irwin, Harvey and Bramwell, Barbara. 1988. "The Devil in Heaven." **Journal of Near-Death Studies** 7(1), 38-43.

Kastenbaum, Robert. 1991. **Death, Society, and Human Experience**. 4th. ed. New York: Macmillan.

Kramer, Kenneth. 1993. **Death Dreams**. New York: Paulist Press.

Kübler-Ross, Elisabeth. 1969. **On Death and Dying**. New York: Macmillan.

Kübler-Ross, Elisabeth. 1983. **On Children and Death**. New York: Macmillan.

Kübler-Ross, Elisabeth. 1987. **AIDS**. New York: Macmillan.

Lindemann, Erich. 1944. "Symptomatology and Management of Acute Grief." **American Journal of Psychiatry** CI, 141-149.

Lindemann, Erich. 1976. "Grief and Grief Management." **The Journal of Pastoral Care** XXX(3), 198-207.

Lindemann, Erich. 1980. "Reactions To One's Own Fatal Illness." **Death: Current Perspectives**, ed. E. Shneidman. 2nd. ed. Palo Alto: Mayfield, 311-319.

Lockhart, Russell. 1977. "Cancer in Myth and Dream." **Spring**, 1-26.

MacMillan, R.L. and Brown, K.W.G. 1982. "Cardiac Arrest Remembered." **A Collection of Near-Death Research Readings** ed. C. Lundahl. Chicago: Nelson-Hall.

Mogenson, Greg. 1992. **Greeting the Angels**. Amityville, NY: Baywood.

Moody, Raymond, A., Jr. 1975. **Life After Life**. Atlanta: Mockingbird Books.

Moody, Raymond, A., Jr. 1988. **The Light Beyond**. New York: Bantam Books.

Morse, Melvin with Perry, Paul. 1990. **Closer to the Light**. New York: Villard Books.

Morse, Melvin with Perry, Paul. 1992. **Transformed by the Light**. New York: Villard Books.

Myers, Frederic, W.H. 1903/1954. **Human Personality and its Survival of Bodily Death**. 2 vols. New York: Longman, Green.

Myers, Frederic, W.H. 1893/1961. **Fragments of Inner Life**. London: The Society for Psychical Research.

Noll, Peter. 1990. **In the Face of Death**, trans. H. Noll. New York: Penguin Books.

Norton, Janice. 1963. "Treatment of a Dying Patient." **The Psychoanalytic Study of a Child** XVIII. New York: International Universities Press, 541-560.

Noyes, Russell, Jr. 1972. "The Experience of Dying." **Psychiatry** 35(2), 174-184.

Noyes, Russell, Jr. 1979. "Near-Death Experiences: Their Interpretation and Significance." **Between Life & Death**, ed. R. Kastenbaum. New York: Springer.

Noyes, Russell, Jr. and Kletti, Roy. 1982. "Depersonalization in the Face of Life-Threatening Danger." **A Collection of Near-Death Research Readings**, ed. C. Lundahl. Chicago: Nelson-Hall.

Osis, Karlis and Haraldsson, Erlendur. 1977. **At the Hour of Death**. New York: Avon Books.

Owens, J.E., Cook, E.W., Stevenson, I. 1990. "Features of 'Near-Death Experience' in Relation to Whether or not Patients were Near Death." **The Lancet** 336 (Nov. 10), 1175-1177.

Oyler, Chris. 1990. **Go Toward the Light**. New York: New American Library.

Pfister, Oskar. 1930/1981. "Shock Thoughts and Fantasies in Extreme Mortal Danger," trans. R. Kletti and R. Noyes, Jr. **Essence** 5(1), 5-20.

Rees, Dewi. 1975. "The Bereaved and their Hallucinations." **Bereavement**, ed. B. Schoenberg. New York: Columbia University Press, 66-71.

Ring, Kenneth. 1980. **Life at Death**. New York: Coward, McCann, & Geoghegan.

Ring, Kenneth. 1984. **Heading Toward Omega**. New York: William Morrow.

Sabom, Michael. 1982. **Recollections of Death**. New York: Harper & Row.

Sato, Koji. 1964. "Death of Zen Masters." **Psychologia** 7, 143-147.

Serdahely, William. 1989-1990. "A Pediatric Near-Death Experience." **Omega** 20(1), 55-62.

Serdahely, William. 1990. "Letter to the Editor." **Omega** 21(3), 249-250.

Sontag, Susan. 1978. **Illness as Metaphor**. New York: Farrar, Straus and Giroux.

von Franz, Marie-Louise. 1987. **On Dreams and Death**, trans. E. Kennedy and V. Brooks. Boston: Shambhala.

Weisman, Avery. 1974. **The Realization of Death**. New York: Jason Aronson.

Weisman, Avery and Hackett, T. 1961. "Predilection to Death." **Psychosomatic Medicine** XXIII (3), 232-256.

Wheelwright, Jane. 1981. **The Death of a Woman**. New York: St. Martin's Press.

Zaleski, Carol. 1987. **Otherworld Journeys**. New York: Oxford University Press.

IV. SOURCES IN THE HISTORY OF IDEAS

Ariès, Philippe. 1981. **The Hour of Our Death**, trans. H. Weaver. New York: Alfred A. Knopf.

Berry, Thomas. 1981. "Dostoevsky and Spiritualism." **Dostoevsky Studies** 2, 43-49.

Boase, T.S.R. 1972. **Death in the Middle Ages.** New York: McGraw-Hill.

Burke, Edmund. 1969. "Dostoevsky's Pulmonary Disease." **Minnesota Medicine** (April), 685-687.

Cohen, Kathleen. 1973. **Metamorphosis of a Death Symbol**. Berkeley: University of California Press.

Dodds, E.R. 1971. "Supernormal Phenomena in Classical Antiquity." **Proceedings of the Society for Psychical Research** Vol. 55. Pt. 203, 189-237.

Dostoevsky, Fyodor. 1936. **The Possessed**, trans. C. Garnett. New York: The Modern Library.

Dostoevsky, Fyodor. 1958. **The Idiot**, trans. C. Garnett. New York: Bantam Books.

Frank, Joseph. 1983. **Dostoevsky, The Years of Ordeal 1850-1859**. Princeton: Princeton University Press.

Frank, Joseph and Goldstein, David, eds. 1987. **Selected Letters of Fyodor Dostoevsky**, trans. A. MacAndrew. New Brunswick: Rutgers University Press.

Helgeland, John. 1984-1985. "The Symbolism of Death in the Later Middle Ages." **Omega** 15(2), 145-160.

Joly, Robert, ed., trans. 1967. **Hippocrate, Du Régime**. Paris: Budé.

Livy. **From the Founding of the City**, trans. B. Foster. Cambridge: Harvard University Press, 1967.

Rice, James. 1985. **Dostoevsky and the Healing Art**. Ann Arbor: Ardis.

Rudolf, Rainer. 1957. **Ars Moriendi. Von Der Kunst Des Heilsamen Lebens und Sterbens**. Köln: Böhlau Verlag.

Wagner-Simon, T. and Haefely-Grauen, I. 1985. "Die Familie Dostojewskij." **Szondiana** 5(1), 5-41.

V. SOURCES IN THE HISTORY OF RELIGIONS

Benz, Ernst. 1968. **Dreams, Hallucinations, Visions**, trans. T. Spiers. New York: The Swedenborg Foundation.

Bleeker, C.J. 1963. "Die Religiöse Bedeutung Der Brücke." **The Sacred Bridge**. Leiden: E.J. Brill.

Boyce, Mary. 1989. **A Persian Stronghold of Zoroastrianism**. Lanham, MD: University Press of America.

Boyce, Mary. ed., trans. 1990. **Textual Sources for the Study of Zoroastrianism**. Chicago: University of Chicago Press.

Corbin, Henry. 1977. **Spiritual Body and Celestial Earth**, trans. N. Pearson. Princeton: Princeton University Press.

Dinzelbacher, P. 1978. "Die Visionen des Mittelalters." **Zeitschrift für Religions-und Geistesgeschichte** XXX(2), 116-128.

Earhart, H. Byron, ed. 1974. "The Ancient Mythology." **Religion in the Japanese Experience: Sources and Interpretations**. Encino, CA: Dickenson Publishing Co.

Flood, Josephine. 1988. **Archeology of the Dreamtime**. Honolulu: University of Hawaii Press.

Gnoli, Gherardo. 1989. "Iranian Religions." **Religions of Antiquity**, ed. R. Seltzer. New York: Macmillan.

Habicht, Christian. 1969. **Die Inschriften des Asklepieions**. Berlin: Walter de Gruyter.

Hutton, Ronald. 1991. **The Pagan Religions of the Ancient British Isles**. Oxford: Basil Blackwell.

Kamakau, Samuel. 1964. **The People of Old**, trans. M. Pukui, ed. D. Burreie. Honolulu: Bishop Museum Press.

Klimkeit, Hans-Joachim. 1980. "Das Kreuzessymbol in der Zentralasiatischen Religionsbegegnung." **Leben und Tod in den Religionen**, ed. G. Stephenson. Darmstadt: Wissenschaftliche Buchgesellschaft, 61-80.

Knight, Frank, A.G. 1953. "Bridge." **Encyclopedia of Religion and Ethics** I, 848-857.

Lauf, Detlef. 1980. "Im Zeichen Des Grossen Übergangs." **Leben und Tod in den Religionen**, ed. G. Stephenson. Darmstadt: Wissenschaftliche Buchgesellschaft, 81-100.

244

Luck, Georg, ed., trans. 1985. **Arcana Mundi**. Baltimore: The Johns Hopkins University Press.

Marika, Wandjuk. 1980. "Foreword." **Australian Dreaming**, ed. J. Isaacs. Sydney: Landsdowne Press.

Molé, M. 1960. "Daena. Le Pont Cinvat et L'initiation dans le Mazdéisme." **Revue de L'Histoire des Religions** 157, 155-185.

Patch, Howard. 1980. **The Other World**. New York: Octagon Books.

Peebles, Rose. 1923. "The Dry Tree: Symbol of Death." **Vassar Mediaeval Studies**, ed. C. Fiske. New Haven: Yale University Press, 59-79.

Pukui, Mary. 1972. **Nana I Ke Kumu**. Honolulu: Hui Hanai.

Radhakrishnan, S. trans. 1953. **The Principal Upanishads**. New York: Harper & Row.

Radin, Paul. 1970. **The Winnebago Tribe**. Lincoln: University of Nebraska Press.

Smith, Jane and Haddad, Yvonne. 1981. **The Islamic Understanding of Death and Resurrection**. Albany: SUNY Press.

Vogel, C. 1964. "Le Pelerinage Penitentiel," **Revue des Sciences Religieuses** 38, 113-153.

VI.   SOURCES IN PHILOSOPHY

Berdyaev, Nicholas. 1952. **The Beginning and the End**, trans. R. M. French. New York: Harper & Row.

Berdyaev, Nicholas. 1957. **Dostoevsky**, trans. D. Attwater. New York: Meridian Books.

Boehme, Jacob. 1958. **Six Theosophic Points**, trans. J. Earle. Ann Arbor: The University of Michigan Press.

Bohm, David. 1983. **Wholeness and the Implicate Order**. London: Ark.

Borkenau, Franz. 1981. **End and Beginning**, trans. R. Lowenthal. New York: Columbia University Press.

Koyré, Alexandre. 1968. **La Philosophie de Jacob Boehme**. New York: Burt Franklin.

Langer, Susanne. 1967. **Mind: An Essay on Human Feeling**. Vol. I. Baltimore: The Johns Hopkins University Press.

Langer, Susanne. 1972. **Mind: An Essay on Human Feeling**. Vol. II. Baltimore: The Johns Hopkins University Press.

VII. SOURCES IN PSYCHIATRY

Andermann, Eva. 1980. "Multifactorial Inheritance in the Epilepsies." **Advances in Epileptology**, eds. R. Canger, F. Angeleri, and J. Penry. New York: Raven Press.

Bear, David, Freeman, Roy, and Greenberg, Mark. 1984. "Behavioral Alterations in Patients with Temporal Lobe Epilepsy." **Psychiatric Aspects of Epilepsy**, ed. D. Blumer. Washington, D.C.: American Psychiatric Press.

Blumer, Dietrich. 1975. "Psychiatric Considerations in Pain." **The Brain** II, ed. R. Rothman and F. Simeone. Philadelphia: W.B. Saunders.

Blumer, Dietrich. 1984. "The Psychiatric Dimensions of Epilepsy." **Psychiatric Aspects of Epilepsy**, ed. D. Blumer. Washington, D.C.: American Psychiatric Press.

Blumer, Dietrich and Benson, D. Frank. 1982. "Psychiatric Manifestations of Epilepsy." **Psychiatric Aspects of Neurologic Disease** II, ed. D. F. Benson and D. Blumer. New York: Grune & Stratton.

Blumer, Dietrich, Heilbronn, Mary, and Himmelhoch, Jonathan. 1988. "Indications for Carbamazepine in Mental Illness." **Comprehensive Psychiatry** 29(2), 108-122.

Cirignotta, F., Todesco, C. V., and Lugaresi, E. 1980. "Temporal Lobe Epilepsy with Ecstatic Seizures (So-Called Dostoevsky Epilepsy)." **Epilepsia** 21, 705-710.

Gastaut, Henri and Collomb, Henri. 1954. "Étude du Comportement Sexuel chez Les Epileptiques Psychomoteurs." **Annales Médico-Psychologiques** 112. 2(5), 657-696.

Hedri, A. 1963. "Unfall und Schicksal." **Mensch, Schicksal, und Tod**, ed. U. Studer-Salzmann. Bern: Hans Huber.

Himmelhoch, Jonathan. 1984. "Major Mood Disorders Related to Epileptic Changes." **Psychiatric Aspects of Epilepsy**, ed. D. Blumer. Washington, D.C.: American Psychiatric Press.

Hobson, J. Allan. 1988. **The Dreaming Brain**. New York: Basic Books.

Jackson, J. Hughlings. 1931. **Selected Writings**, ed. J. Taylor. Vol. I. London: Hodder and Stoughton.

Jung, Carl. 1960. **The Structure and Dynamics of the Psyche. Collected Works**, trans. R. F. C. Hull. New York: Pantheon Books.

Jung, Carl. 1961. **Memories, Dreams, Reflections**, trans. R. and C. Winston. New York: Random House.

Jung, Carl. 1925/1989. **Analytical Psychology**, ed. W. McGuire. Princeton: Princeton University Press.

Jung, Carl. 1973. **Letters**. Vol. I: 1906-1950, trans. R. F. C. Hull. Princeton: Princeton University Press.

Jung, Carl. 1975. **Letters**. Vol. II: 1951-1961, trans. R. F. C. Hull. Princeton: Princeton University Press.

Lennox, William. 1951. "The Heredity of Epilepsy as Told by Relatives and Twins." **Journal of the American Medical Association** 146(6), 529-536.

Niedermeyer, Ernst. 1984. "Neurologic Aspects of the Epilepsies." **Psychiatric Aspects of Epilepsy**, ed. D. Blumer. Washington, D.C.: American Psychiatric Press.

Riese, Walther. 1958. "The Disease of Vincent van Gogh." **Ciba Symposium** 6(5), 198-205.

Roth, Martin and Harper, Max. 1962. "Temporal Lobe Epilepsy and the Phobic Anxiety-Depersonalization Syndrome. Part II." **Comprehensive Psychiatry** 3(4), 215-225.

Slater Eliot and Beard, A.W. 1963. "The Schizophrenia-like Psychoses of Epilepsy." **The British Journal of Psychiatry**, 109, 95-150.

Szondi, Leopold. 1936. "Der Neurotiker im Lichte der psychoanalytischen, neuro-endokrinen und erbpathologischen Forschungen." **Schweizer Archiv für Neurologie und Psychiatries** 37(2), 313-334.

Szondi, Leopold. 1937. "Contributions to 'Fate Analysis,' An Attempt at a Theory of Choice in Love." **Acta Psychologica** 3(1), 1-80.

Szondi, Leopold. 1939. "Heilpädagogik in der Prophylaxe der Nerven- und Geisteskrankeiten." **Sonderdruck aus dem Bericht über den I. Internationalen Kongress für Heilpädagogik**, 24-61.

Szondi, Leopold. 1949. "Revision der Frage der 'erblichen Belastung.'" **II. Sonderfragen der Medizin**, 1-17.

Szondi, Leopold. 1956. **Ich-Analyse**. Bern: Hans Huber.

Szondi, Leopold. 1960. **Lehrbuch der Experimentellen Triebdiagnostik**. Bern: Hans Huber.

Szondi, Leopold. 1963. **Schicksalsanalytische Therapie**. Bern: Hans Huber.

Szondi, Leopold. 1969. **Kain, Gestalten des Bösen**. Bern: Hans Huber.

Szondi, Leopold. 1972. **Introduction a L'Analyse du Destin**, trans. C. Van Reeth. Louvain: Éditions Nauwelaerts.

Szondi, Leopold. 1973. **Moses, Antwort auf Kain**. Bern: Hans Huber.

Szondi, Leopold. 1977. **Triebpathologie**. Zweite Auflage. Bern: Hans Huber.

Szondi, Leopold. 1980. **Die Triebentmischten**. Bern: Hans Huber.

Szondi, Leopold. 1987. **Schicksalsanalyse**. Vierte Auflage. Bern: Hans Huber.

Szondi, Leopold. 1954/1989. "Glaube als Schicksal." **Szondiana** 9(2), 53-56.

Szondi, Leopold. 1955/1992. "Die Sprachen des Unbewussten." **Szondiana** 12(2), 8-31.

Taylor, David and Marsh, Susan. 1980. "Hughlings Jackson's Dr. Z." **Journal of Neurology, Neurosurgery, and Psychiatry** 43, 758-767.

Temkin, Owsei. 1971. **The Falling Sickness**. 2nd. ed. rev. Baltimore: The Johns Hopkins Press.

Temkin, Owsei and Temkin, C. Lillian. 1968. "Subjective Experiences in Temporal Lobe Epilepsy: An Anonymous Report of 1825." **Bulletin of the History of Medicine** 42, 566-568.

Walker, A. Earl and Blumer, Dietrich. 1984. "Behavioral Effects of Temporal Lobectomy for Temporal Lobe Epilepsy." **Psychiatric Aspects of Epilepsy**, ed. D. Blumer. Washington, D.C.: American Psychiatric Press.

Vogel, Paul. 1935. "Joh. Purkinjes Auffassung der Epilepsie." **Nervenarzt** 8, 228-232.

VIII. SOURCES IN PSYCHOLOGY

Bürgi-Meyer, Karl. 1987. "Das familiäre Unbewusste nach Leopold Szondi im Lichte Transpersonaler Psychologie." **Szondiana** 7(2), 5-24.

Dajer, Tony. 1992. "Divided Selves." **Discover** (Sept.), 38-44, 69.

248

Ferenczi, Sandor. 1921. "Die Symbolik der Brücke." **Internationale Zeitschrift für Psychoanalyse** 7, 211-213.

Ferenczi, Sandor. 1922. "Die Brückensymbolik und die Don Juan-Legende." **Internationale Zeitschrift für Psychoanalyse** 3, 77-78.

Freud, Sigmund. 1953. **The Interpretation of Dreams**. Standard **Edition**. Vol. IV.

Freud, Sigmund. 1957. "The Unconscious." **Standard Edition. Vol. XIV**, 166-195.

Freud, Sigmund. 1957a. "Thoughts for the Times on War and Death." **Standard Edition**. Vol. XIV, 279-297.

Freud, Sigmund. 1958. "A Note on the Unconscious in Psychoanalysis." **Standard Edition**. Vol. XII, 260-264.

Freud, Sigmund. 1959. "Mourning and Melancholia." **Collected Papers**, trans. J. Riviere. Vol. IV. New York: Basic Books.

Freud, Sigmund. 1958. "The Theme of the Three Caskets." **Standard Edition**. Vol. XII, 292-301.

Hughes, Richard. 1992. **Return of the Ancestor**. New York: Peter Lang.

Jaffè, Aniela. 1963. **Apparitions and Precognition**. New Hyde Park, NY: University Books.

MacDonald, W. Scott and Oden, Chester. 1977. "*Aumakua*: Behavioral Direction Visions in Hawaiians." **Journal of Abnormal Psychology** 86(2), 189-194.

Murphy, Gardner and Ballou, Robert, eds. 1960. **William James on Psychical Research**. New York: Viking.

Persinger, Michael. 1987. **Neuropsychological Bases of God Beliefs**. New York: Praeger.

Reimbold, Ernst. 1972. "Die Brücke als Symbol." **Symbolon I**, 55-78.

Thompson, C. 1982. "*Anwesenheit*: Psychopathology and Clinical Associations." **British Journal of Psychiatry** 141, 628-630.

Ullman, Montague and Krippner, Stanley. 1973. **Dream Telepathy**. New York: Macmillan.

Wilder, Thornton. 1928. **The Bridge of San Louis Rey**. New York: Grosset and Dunlap.

Witztum, Eliezer, Greenberg, David and Buchbinder, Jacob. 1990. "A Very Narrow Bridge." **Psychotherapy** 27(1) (Spring), 124-131.

IX. SOURCES IN THEOLOGY

Augustine, Saint. **The City of God**, trans. P. Levine. The Loeb Classical Library.

Gatch, Milton, McC. 1969. "Some Theological Reflections on Death from the Early Church Through the Reformation." **Perspectives on Death**, ed. L. Mills. Nashville: Abingdon Press, 99-136.

Gregory the Great, Saint. 1959. **Dialogues**, trans. O. Zimmerman. New York: Fathers of the Church.

Hughes, Richard. 1982. "Bereavement and Pareschatology." **Encounter** 43(4), 361-375.

"Ignatius to the Ephesians." **The Apostolic Fathers**. Cambridge: Harvard University Press, 1970.

"Ignatius to the Romans." **The Apostolic Fathers**. Cambridge: Harvard University Press, 1970.

Kerr, Hugh. 1943. **A Compend of Luther's Theology**. Philadelphia: Westminster.

Le Goff, Jacques. 1984. **The Birth of Purgatory**, trans. A. Goldhammer. Chicago: University of Chicago Press.

Luther, Martin. **Lectures on Genesis. Luther's Works**. Vols. 5, 6.

Luther, Martin. **Lectures on Romans. Luther's Works**. Vol. 25.

Luther, Martin. "A Sermon on Preparing to Die, 1519." **Luther's Works**. Vol. 42.

Meinhold, Peter. 1980. "Leben und Tod im Urteil des Christentums." **Leben und Tod in den Religionen**, ed. G. Stephenson. Darmstadt: Wissenschaftliche Buchgesellschaft, 144-164.

Miller, Arlene. 1970. "The Theologies of Luther and Boehme in the Light of Their *Genesis* Commentaries." **Harvard Theological Review** 63, 261-303.

Miller-McLemore, Bonnie. 1988. **Death, Sin, and the Mortal Life**. Atlanta: Scholars Press.

Oberman, Heiko. 1992. **Luther**, trans. E. Walliser-Schwarzbart. New York: Image Books.

Pauck, Wilhelm and Pauck, Marion. 1976. **Paul Tillich**. Vol. I: Life. New York: Harper & Row.

Petersen, Joan. 1984. **The *Dialogues* of Gregory the Great in Their Late Antique Cultural Background**. Toronto: Pontifical Institute of Mediaeval Studies.

Rosenwein, Barbara. 1971. "Feudal War and Monastic Peace." **Viator** 2, 129-157.

Steidle, Basilius. 1971. "Die Kosmische Vision des Gottesmannes Benedikt (1)." **Erbe und Auftrag** 47, 187-192, 298-315, 409-414.

Tauler, Johannes. **Vom Gottförmigen Menschen**, ed. F. Noerr. Stuttgart: Reclam, 1961.

Tillich, Hannah. 1973. **From Time to Time**. New York: Stein and Day.

Tillich, Paul. 1948. **The Shaking of the Foundations**. New York: Charles Scribner's Sons.

Tillich, Paul. 1955. **The New Being**. New York: Charles Scribner's Sons.

Tillich, Paul. 1969. "That They May Have Life." **Union Seminary Quarterly Review** XX(1), 3-8.

INDEX

DATE DUE			
MAY 12 1992			
			Printed in USA